Nursing Supervision

Nursing Supervision

A Guide for Clinical Practice

Stephen Power

SAGE Publications
London • Thousand Oaks • New Delhi

SAGE Publications Ltd
6 Bonhill Street
London EC2A 4PU

SAGE Publications Inc.
2455 Teller Road
Thousand Oaks, California 91320

SAGE Publications India Pvt Ltd
32, M-Block Market
Greater Kailash – I
New Delhi 110 048

British Library Cataloguing in Publication data

A catalogue record for this book is available
from the British Library

ISBN 0 7619 6007 4
ISBN 0 7619 6008 2 (pbk)

Library of Congress catalog record available

Typeset by Mayhew Typesetting, Rhayader, Powys
Printed in Great Britain by Biddles Ltd, Guildford, Surrey

*Dedicated, with love, to Molly and
Ken, my first supervisors, and to Ian
my first, and life-long, supervisee*

Contents

Acknowledgements

I was once advised that when someone says 'I would like to write a book', it can be a desire expressed in the language of enthusiastic ignorance and that the astute would-be author is more apt to say: 'I would like to *have written* a book'. Having been embroiled in writing this, my first, book for more than a year, I am absolutely clear about the subtle difference in those two statements – and the wisdom of that advice. I have also discovered that even if yours is the only name to appear on the cover, it is virtually impossible to write a book without involving other people. Here, I want to say 'thank you' to those people who allowed me to not only indulge my enthusiastically ignorant desire to write a book, but also helped me to know what it finally feels like to *have* written one.

This book would not have happened at all without Sage Publications and I owe much to Susan Worsey who was brave enough to offer me a contract, in the first place. Also at Sage, Melissa Dunlop has been my editorial 'rock' at times of confusion, desperation and layout-crisis. Philip Barker and Gary Winship read the original proposal and offered me the benefit of their experience. Derek Farrell also read the proposal and about half of the chapters in draft form. His astute comments, enthusiasm and friendship have been extremely valuable. Peter Wilkin was kind enough to read and comment upon Chapter 5, *twice*, and also let me reproduce some of his work on contracting and his views on the supervisor/supervisee relationship.

The section on group supervision owes much to my own work with five Nurse-Fellows at Canterbury Christ Church University College, namely: Julie Johnstone, Fiona McArthur-Rouse, Sue Simmons, Mark Wilbourn and Anneliese Willis who offered me their thoughts on the value of group supervision processes. I am also indebted to Professor Bill Lemmer, Head of the Department of Mental Health and Learning Disabilities, who has constantly demonstrated his pragmatic support for my writing.

My friends Mohammad Abuel-Ealeh, Richard Barrett, Tommy Donovan and Karen Worden have all offered their support and listened to my troubles before and throughout this entire project. Strangely enough, they have remained my friends. I am sure that says more about them than it does about me. Dr Paul Dickinson was my first 'proper' supervisor when I entered the world of clinical psychotherapy, in 1984, and I am grateful for all that he taught me and the fact that I now also call him my friend.

Introduction: Me, clinical supervision, nurses and this book

When Stephen met supervision

I was a mental health nurse, with over ten years' experience, before I had ever heard of clinical supervision. The consultant psychiatrist in whose team I worked was developing the practice of psychodynamic psychotherapy within his catchment area, and I wanted to be involved. Although it was psychotherapy, and not supervision, that I was interested in, one is inextricably linked to the other and I quickly learnt the first 'rule' of psychotherapy – no supervision, no practice. Whether I wanted it or not, my clinical supervision experience had begun.

It was difficult at first, and sometimes even downright unpleasant. For starters, I doubt that I would have agreed to meet with some extremely skilled colleagues late on Friday evenings, always off-duty and unpaid to discuss my caseload for any other reasons than that I wanted to practise psychotherapy and that such meetings came with the work. I had a sense of feeling out-of-my-depth in my first supervision group and frequently mentally 'rehearsed' almost every word I uttered and then often wished that I had kept silent.

My second problem was that the hard-bitten community nurses, with whom I shared an open-plan office, found my willingness to drive fifteen miles in the opposite direction to my home, at the end of a long week, puzzling in the least. Walking past their desks I would encounter a series of confused faces, shrugging shoulders and shaking heads that often left me doubting my own actions. But things change and as my psychotherapy work developed, supervision became an indispensable experience. The more clinical work

I did, the more I needed supervision and the more supervision I received the better my practice became and the less my colleagues frowned and shrugged as I left for supervision.

Since those first tentative steps, my experience of clinical supervision, both as a supervisee and as a supervisor, has been extensive in nursing and other areas of health care. I am still excited about being involved in what I see as a pivotal aspect of clinical nursing and one that should not be restricted to small pockets of nurses working with very specialised techniques.

The point of this book

A major problem during my early supervision experiences, was that no one ever told me *how* to be supervised. I was offered no theories or models of supervision and there was no formal training available for the supervisors. Supervision simply happened around me as I watched what everyone else did and tried, sometimes vainly, to follow suit. When I began to supervise others, in the absence of any formal training and information, I relied on using the communication skills I honed through talking to patients and the knowledge and experiences I had acquired through being supervised. In fact, it is only very recently that there has been a recognition of the need to define the specific and distinct skills, personal characteristics and practical considerations necessary to perform (and receive) clinical supervision effectively.

Clinical supervision, at least in nursing, is still in its early childhood – if not infancy – and many nurses who want to become involved in this important extension to their clinical practice, simply do not know how or where to start. This book is for all nurses who are curious, or confused, about the nitty-gritty, practical and real-life aspects of clinical supervision. I have focused on what they will need to do, and think about, in order to begin practising or receiving clinical supervision within any nursing organisation. This book is also for those clinical nurse supervisors and supervisees who may have started down this exciting road, and are now wondering what it is they need to do and think about in order to keep going or, perhaps, even bring their supervision experience to a satisfactory conclusion.

It was not my intention to write an academic thesis on clinical supervision and I have no high ideals to win grand prizes for theoretical postulation. I have only ever wanted to write a book that can be *used*, in real and practical ways, by any nurse to whom clinical supervision is even remotely relevant. I have since discovered that it is virtually impossible to offer valid and relevant information without some reference to academic text and theorising to a certain extent and, therefore, I have offered some discussion of models and theories of clinical supervision, hopefully in an accessible and thought-provoking way.

I strongly believe in the potential of clinical supervision to enhance nursing practice and it should not be difficult to discern my positive bias on reading the book. However, as with most things in life, there is a potential for clinical supervision to be misused or abused, and, because of this, I have not shied away from describing some difficulties and problems that can arise in the course of supervision practice. I hope that, overall, my views will be seen as balanced and the inclusion of the challenging aspects of clinical supervision as instructive, rather than destructive.

I am tempted to suggest that the purpose of this book is to *teach* or to *advise* or to *enlighten* or to *guide* and if any reader feels that I have achieved those objectives I will certainly be extremely pleased. However, my real purpose in writing this book is, to *encourage*. I hope to encourage thinking about the value and purpose of clinical supervision by nurses new to the concept, and discussions on how to begin the practice of supervision by those nurses who have previously given thought to its benefits. I also want to encourage awareness of the potential pitfalls that supervisors and supervisees can encounter in order that practitioners do what they can to avoid them.

The principles underlining this book

My teaching, in nurse education, is guided by the principle that what I do within a given time-slot, will always be inadequate. Even when I leave seemingly satisfied students, I am clear that there could have been more to say, another exercise to perform, or another slide to present to them that would have increased their understanding and knowledge. I have used a similar principle in writing this book and I am convinced that even if I had written more words, produced more diagrams and offered different content, that there would still be readers who would have preferred other issues to be addressed or that I had chosen other ways to address them. And I would have to agree with them.

Over the years I have evolved a style of teaching that allows me to be myself – and as real as possible – in the lecture-room. As it, generally, 'works' for my students, I saw no reason to change that approach, and so readers will find much of 'me' in here. Therefore, throughout the book, I have tried to write as I try to teach: mixing together what I hope will be a palatable blend of factual information, opinion, academic theory, anecdotal material, serious comment, tables, diagrams, and good-humoured banter and thought-provoking exercises. I hope it works for you, too.

Using the exercises

The exercises, found in the 'Think About . . .' boxes, in each chapter, are an essential aspect of the book. The intention of these exercises is, not surprisingly, to make the reader think – and perhaps feel – a little more about the topic being discussed in the main body of the text. Because most of the exercises require the reader to make personal responses I felt that it would be confusing to offer a set of 'right answers' to the exercises. In most cases, there *are* no right answers and what readers decide for themselves, on completion of each exercise, will often be of most importance. Astute readers will, however, find that some of the exercise questions also contain my thoughts on typical responses to certain situations. If these do not fit their own, they may at least be a starting point for further thinking and debate. I would suggest that the exercises can be used individually, for quiet contemplation, or as the basis for discussion in pairs and small groups, perhaps as part of clinical supervision trainings or work groups. Some readers may prefer to carry out the exercises with pen and paper handy, to make notes, while others may simply wish to give thought to them. Whatever way readers choose to carry out the exercises, the essential ingredient to making them work will probably be nothing more than a little time.

The terminology in this book

For the sake of clarity, I have chosen to use only one word or phrase to describe those people or 'things' that frequently have several guises in the modern nursing world. I am aware that there is a chance I may offend those readers who do not agree with my descriptors, but they are offered in the hope that my intention to facilitate understanding through simplification will be widely accepted, even when my 'labels' are not.

In this book, 'nurses' are all those people who have attained a recognised professional qualification in nursing, no matter what specialism. It includes, for my purposes, midwives and health visitors. 'Patient' describes everyone that may come into contact with a nurse for the purpose of receiving nursing care. The term 'nursing care' signifies everything that a nurse can legitimately do to, with or for, a patient, in the course of his professional life. 'The nursing organisation' is the phrase that I have chosen to describe all of the possible places where nurses may provide nursing care to patients. Throughout the book, readers should have little difficulty in deciding where this 'label' is being used in a 'micro' way (to describe wards, units, day hospitals, etc.) or in a 'macro' way (to describe large departments, divisions, trusts and health authorities, etc.). 'Supervisor', 'clinical supervisor' and 'clinical nurse supervisor' are used interchangeably to describe the qualified nurse that offers clinical supervision to other nurses.

Although I have tried to limit my use of anything other than 'supervisor', I have used the longer phrases, to offer greater understanding as I felt necessary. The phrases 'supervisee' and 'clinical supervisee' are used to describe any qualified nurse who is receiving supervision from a clinical supervisor. I have tried to limit myself, particularly in the body of the text, to using the phrase 'supervision' to describe the coming together of supervisor and a supervisee but there are times when I have used 'clinical supervision' and 'clinical supervision for nurses' – especially in titles and subtitles – because I felt it might offer increased understanding. All clinical supervisors are assigned female gender and all supervisees, male. It barely needs me to explain that the situation is different, and probably less simple, in real life. Once again, my intention for doing this is to achieve clarity through simplification and the designations were made arbitrarily.

1
Nurses and Supervision – Myths, Trouble and Misconceptions

Key issues in this chapter

- The myth of nurses as angels
- Why the term 'clinical supervision' may be obsolete
- Common misconceptions of clinical supervision
- Why nurses may avoid clinical supervision

The myth of nurses – angels from heaven and hell

I have been called many things in my life, but I doubt that anyone would ever mistake me for an angel. My stocky masculine build, severely receding hairline, gruff Northern accent and general demeanour is likely to suggest something quite different to the unsuspecting 'person-in-the-street' meeting me for the first time. But what impression might have been given if only my professional reputation had gone before me? What if a mutual friend had mentioned me, with nothing more than my professional credentials to prepare the ground? What might the third person have made of the following introduction:

> My friend has been a nurse since 1973, starting as a cadet at the age of sixteen, mostly making tea and running errands. After qualifying, my friend worked in a variety of challenging areas, including acute psychiatry, forensic nursing, community nursing and psychotherapy. My friend has given all of his working life to the care of others, either by nursing them directly – sometimes not without some personal risk – and, more recently, by helping to teach other people to nurse the mentally ill.

How conceivable is it that the listener's immediate response to that introduction of me, might be something like:
'Your friend deserves a medal!'
Or: 'Your friend must be a very special person!'
Or: 'People can't learn to do that sort of thing, they are born to it!'
Or: 'Your friend must be a true Angel of Mercy!'
Whatever the comment passed would be, I am certain that the seeds of any myth surrounding my potential as a guiding spirit with wings and a halo, that might have germinated from those first few isolated words of introduction, would soon find themselves on more fallow ground, a few moments after the *real me* turned up.

A huge problem for nurses is that, as a profession, we are regularly subjected to the sort of erroneous 'labelling' that can cause us to fall into the trap of having to behave like super – if not supernatural – beings. The myth of nurses as 'angels' is constantly perpetuated through the media. Television drama, film and newspapers regularly – and sometimes even when the allusion is intended to be ironic – invest nurses with an ethereal quality that is frequently relevant neither to the work nurses do nor to the actual qualities that they possess as *real* people. The victim of a land-mine explosion described his first moments of consciousness after waking up in hospital, in this way: '. . . (there was) a bright light shining in my face – all I could see were two blonde nurses in white, they looked like angels' (*The Times*, 29 March 1997). It is not difficult to understand why this unfortunate man used that particular analogy to describe his situation. Having awakened to the sight of two women, both wearing white and with their blonde hair haloed by a bright light and perhaps seeing both women with (presumably) compassionate expressions on their faces, he could well be forgiven for assuming that he had died and gone to heaven. His comments are to my mind, though, typical of the generally fabulous esteem in which nurses are held by the public. The angelic metaphor is, however, often one that is rejected by nurses themselves. Rather than becoming a coveted appellation, the label of 'Angel of Mercy' has become to be regarded by some nurses as a convenient stick to beat them with. One staff nurse, remonstrating in the British Press about how the government's attitude to paying nurses may have affected their morale stated: 'Every year they kick us in the teeth. They won't mind is the attitude – they are angels' (*The Guardian*, 7 February, 1997).

Occasionally, some nurses demonstrate that there are those amongst the numbers of earthly 'angels' who are not only human, but are also incapable of behaving within the professional, moral and legal codes that separate the angels from the devils; the worthy from the untrustworthy; and the unrecognised, but exceptional, nurses from the infamous patient-killers. When nurses make the headlines for the *wrong* reasons – and, thankfully, it remains a relatively rare occurrence – the myth of nurses as angels is often given a new lease of life, albeit from a much less sympathetic position. The general public, usually via the press and the courts, express their abject confusion about just *how* these infallible corporeal manifestations of all that is good and who – almost to a *woman* – never strike, swear, smoke or have sex outside marriage, can possibly fall from the very high pedestal on which they have been placed by the general public.

When nurses are seen to fail in the eyes of the public, however, they are usually seen to fail badly, and in a way that causes people to feel seriously let down and disappointed in them. As an example of this, I offer the comments made by a barrister prosecuting a nurse accused of committing grievous bodily harm on patients, who described the case as being primarily about: '. . . betrayal'. The barrister also told the court that nurses: 'enjoy a very high place in the hearts of the public – they are deemed caring, devoted angels of mercy' (*The Guardian*, 4 October 1996).

The general view of nurses as angels (and sometimes as 'fallen angels') is not one that is likely to go away overnight, if ever. Whether nurses favour the angelic association or not, they are pretty much stuck with it, and perhaps also stuck in a difficult no-win situation. When nurses try to reject the public's view of them as the personification of perfection, they leave themselves wide open to charges of false modesty and confirmation that, as a group, they lack a strong enough sense of self-worth necessary to bring about longed-for changes in their professional standing. Unfortunately, the argument that nurses are only human can be quickly turned against them and into a reason why they are sometimes viewed as the medical world's second-class citizens, undeserving of higher pay and better working conditions. If, on the other hand, nurses try to live up to the myth of themselves as the indefatigable purveyors of compassion and care, they are, again, ultimately bound to lose the argument. No one is tirelessly perfect or constantly capable of caring with no thought for themselves. A strong argument against clinical supervision is that nurses do not need it and can quite happily work day in and day out without support – or caring – for themselves. Supporters of that view, may well have bought in to this second argument. They may, indeed, have accepted the myth of nurses, themselves. Similar to the way in which some comedians feel that it is acceptable to make jokes about their own culture, I feel that I have a right to express my view of nurses. It is this: nurses are special people but nurses are not, nor ever will be angels. When nurses try to live up to the popular ideal of themselves as super-beings they immediately become open to failure and disenchantment. Nurses are, fortunately, not super-beings but human beings with all the faults, failings and foibles of any other person. To seek support and guidance for what we do at work is human behaviour that, I believe, should not be discouraged or undermined. This book is primarily about why this myth of nurses needs to be shattered – and sooner rather than later. For nurses' sakes.

The trouble with supervision

Supervision is a confusing and troublesome concept. Just say the word to some nurses and they will be instantly reminded of traumatic training experiences of threatening senior staff standing over them, ever-watchful, ever-critical. Nurses are well-trained; competent, busy professionals who have committed all of their available time and energy to the care and treatment of the patient. As a group, nurses have demonstrated their professional responsibility time and time again; and the few rotten apples are generally discarded from the barrel, soon enough. Nurses wouldn't be nurses if they wanted to spend time on themselves, would they? Why waste valuable time and money on something that doesn't help deal with the problems that the job throws at nurses every day?

It may even seem like double standards to train people to a level where they are capable of dealing with a myriad of complex tasks and stressful situations, and then not expect them to cope without constant supervision from a more experienced colleague.

To compound the confusion, nurses are very busy people whose limited time is, by necessity, given almost exclusively to the care and consideration of *other* people. Treating and caring for patients is the main reason nurses come to work every day and often go home satisfied, if exhausted. Without patients there would be no reason for the nurse to be there at all, and certainly nothing worthwhile for them to do. So, surely, it makes perfect sense to allocate all of the time available to this purpose?

In addition, the idea of being supervised, as a nurse, has too often become associated with – at worst – ideas of incompetence and – at best – the implicit suggestion that, one day when you have been deemed good enough, you will be able to carry out this procedure without being observed (or *supervised*). It is hardly surprising, then, that those who have been subjected to that sort of negative experience as students will be wary of exposing themselves to something similar as qualified staff. Surely the point of being qualified is that the nurse is considered capable of getting on with the job without the need for intrusive and unnecessary observation from other qualified staff?

What's in a name?

A big problem that clinical supervision has, is the name itself. The word 'supervision' is enough to put people off before they ever meet with their supervisor. It stands to reason that if something sounds unpleasant, the expected human reaction would be to avoid it. Who, for example, would want to have 'Swedish massage', for aching limbs, if it was called '*having someone pummel your back with their bare knuckles*'? Well OK, each to their own pleasures, but I guess that the majority of people would say that the latter description *sounds* less attractive.

Unfortunately, perhaps, there are a number of definitions of the word 'supervision' that do nothing to allay anxieties that it might be, on the whole, an unpleasant experience. The *Collins Universal English Dictionary* (1987) puts the metaphorical boot in by taking the no-frills approach to 'supervision' by describing it as: 'The act of over-seeing or directing work'. Leddick and Bernard (1980) take a similarly hard line by confirming that clinical supervisors are expected to over-see the work of another and to often carry responsibility for the quality of that work. This alone would probably be enough to put many experienced nurses off the idea, but it gets even worse. By way of confirmation of the hierarchical relationship inherent in supervision, Williams (1992) comments that anyone designated as a supervisor is often seen as the 'boss', the person who is to be obeyed and who tells us what to do and is responsible for our actions.

Evans (1997), has pointed out that there is an intrinsically authoritarian feel to the phrase, which has been masked, in some cases, by the use of more user-friendly language, such as *mentoring* and *facilitation*. I would add other offenders to the list of 'let's call a spade a manual ground-improving implement' words including: preceptoring, consulting and guided reflection. The real problem is that the more words we use to *avoid* the one that we have – and should be using – the more we dig a bigger hole for ourselves, with that 'ground-improving implement'. The solution is, I suggest, to stick to the words we have and be clear about what they mean and, just as importantly, what they do not mean. In the next section I want to offer my views on what the words 'clinical supervision for nurses' should *not* imply.

Three common misconceptions of clinical supervision

As with so many areas of life, a little understanding can be a dangerous thing; and supervision and how it is perceived by nurses is no exception. The potentially positive, useful and even desirable qualities it possesses are given a negative twist, either because they are seen in isolation from each other or perhaps because it is safer to decry something that we do not fully understand.

I will take three major misconceptions of supervision that have grown out of the corruption of its more positive and desirable intentions.

MISCONCEPTION 1 – HAVE YOUR JOB EXPLAINED TO YOU!
The supervisor is the expert when it comes to clinical nursing practice and will always have better ideas than you, the supervisee. The supervisor is the only person capable of nursing anyone properly and if you don't do it the supervisor's way, you are doing it wrong! Right?

Not really! A crucial misconception about supervision is that it is where you go to be told how to do your job properly. We can all benefit from new ideas, advice and suggestions, but to say that the supervisee has everything to learn about her work and nothing of value to currently offer the patients would be insulting at best, and, at worst, potentially dangerous.

It can be argued that two heads may be at least as good as one and that supervision may be a place where someone can learn more about how best to practise nursing. It must also be remembered that supervision has the potential to cause the supervisee to become *de-skilled*, even before they arrive for the first session. Prospective supervisees will be easily discouraged by an emphasis on the educational potential of supervision – which in itself can be very professionally rejuvenating – if it coincides with an idea, however covert, that the supervisory relationship will be akin to that of a university professor struggling to educate a pre-GCSE student.

MISCONCEPTION 2 – HAVE YOUR HEAD EXAMINED!
Clinical nursing supervision is solely concerned with supporting the nurse from a personal perspective, in a way that is more appropriately associated with therapy or counselling than the practice of nursing.

Some nursing authors, including Faugier (1996), have raised this second, important misconception of supervision, which because it has a more positive undertone, is perhaps generally more widely accepted by the majority of nurses as a legitimate aspect of supervision.

However, ultimately, it is just as damaging and off-putting as the first misconception, due to its narrow focus and implicit emphasis on the nurse's failings and weaknesses. There is nothing fundamentally wrong with the suggestion that nurses should be supported in their work, even from the perspective of how the job affects them, personally and emotionally. A problem arises when prospective supervisees connect the idea of receiving supervision directly with the notion of having their heads – and personalities – examined by a supervisor who may want to practise their six-week basic counselling skills training on them.

MISCONCEPTION 3 – BE WARNED!
Nursing supervision is closely allied to the appraisal process and has a primary function of making sure that the nurse is legal, ethical, honest, decent and obeying orders at all times.

It is unfortunate, especially for those intent on encouraging nurses to savour the benefits of supervision that, traditionally, the third essential functional strand it has to offer has been described as that of managerial in nature. This is exactly the sort of language that causes experienced nurses to scream 'don't tell me how to manage my patients', as they storm out of the supervisory session never to return.

There are areas of health care – social work, midwifery and others – where the term managerial supervision can sometimes mean having work scrutinised by a senior colleague, often a line-manager who has the capacity to take disciplinary action, with the intention of ensuring that certain agreed goals are met.

Some nurses have been given to understand, in some instances by their nurse managers, that the managerial function in clinical nursing supervision is also linked to appraisal, Individual Performance Review (IPR) and the disciplinary procedure. I have known supervision to be used as a way of punishing or controlling nurses who are considered to have performed below standard. I have also seen it used as a method of allowing unit or locality managers to 'over-see' the work of ten nurses by talking to one clinical supervisor every few weeks. It is hardly surprising, then, that nurses are reluctant to engage in what may really be just another form of managerial scrutiny, thinly disguised as 'professional development'.

A case of clinical supervision

Sarah is a mental health nurse with eleven years' post-qualification experience. Her post-registration qualifications include a diploma in Community Mental Health Nursing (ENB 812), a recordable qualification in Psychodynamic Techniques for Registered Mental Health Nurses (ENB 660), and a formal training in systemic family therapy at a widely recognised training centre in London. She is employed as senior clinical nurse specialist in psychotherapy within a local Hospital Trust in the north of England and is based at a community mental health centre.

In addition to her managerial and administrative responsibilities Sarah currently manages a clinical caseload of twelve once-weekly individual clients, two once-weekly psychodynamic psychotherapy groups and once-weekly attendance at the Trust's family therapy clinic, where she is currently facilitating the therapy of one family and supporting the work of other therapists with two more families. Sarah also clinically supervises the work of six other health professionals – three nurse therapists, two social workers and a clinical psychologist – all of whom are practising psychodynamically-orientated therapies.

Despite her experience and seniority, Sarah receives clinical supervision for each of the main areas of her clinical practice. She meets with the consultant psychiatrist on a weekly basis (for 1 hour) to discuss her 'individual' psychotherapy work, rotating the discussion of her caseload so that every patient has been discussed with her supervisor at least once in every calendar month. Sarah also meets weekly (for 1½ hours) with two other nurses to discuss the psychotherapy groups that she conducts. This meeting is facilitated by an experienced and trained group therapy supervisor, who ensures that the three supervisees each have regular (and fairly equal) supervision time, by rotating the order of presentations to the group. When Sarah attends on a week that she is not due to present one of her own groups for discussion, she is encouraged by the supervisor to offer suggestions and constructive comments on the work of the other nurses. Finally, Sarah also meets fortnightly with the two other nurses facilitating family therapy, to discuss their work and offer each other support and guidance for this specialist activity.

Sarah is very clear that such regular and formal clinical supervision is a major part of the reason for her widely recognised professional status and clinical competence. She doubts that she would be able to continue working in any of the specialist fields she does, currently, without the time spent in formal reflection on the processes and consequences of her work.

Think about . . . having too much of a good thing!

Even dyed-in-the-wool supervision fans would possibly accept that there is a point where clinical practice could become overshadowed – if not totally obliterated – by the necessity for almost constant attendance at supervision sessions. Having read the fictional, yet clinically accurate, vignette of Sarah's supervisory experience address the following questions.

1 Do you consider the amount of clinical supervision Sarah is subject to, as excessive?
2 Given Sarah's experience and current role, do you think she should be supervised for her own work, at all?
3 Do you agree that Sarah should be supervised by the clinicians (particularly the non-nurses) mentioned in the extract? If not, who would be the most appropriate professional to supervise the various aspects of her work?

Personal reasons to avoid clinical supervision

There are a number of reasons why many nurses may extol the virtues of supervision, perhaps in discussion with colleagues or even through their writings in professional journals, and still find it difficult to sit down in front of a supervisor and talk about their clinical work. Although it may appear something of a paradox, what I am suggesting is that the prospective supervisee may often avoid supervision because he is afraid of what might happen to him when he gets there, without actually being aware that he is avoiding it for that reason.

Some reasons why nurses may wish to avoid becoming personally involved in clinical supervision, while simultaneously expressing a positive appreciation of its benefits, can include:

- A dread of being dis-empowered by the supervisor.
- A fear of being threatened by a more skilful colleague (supervisor).
- An uneasiness around admitting professional shortcomings and lack of knowledge.
- Concerns about being rejected as inadequate, or inferior.
- Anxieties around being overwhelmed by the problems of the work being discussed.
- Misgivings about becoming dependent upon the supervisor.
- Worries connected to becoming emotionally distressed, angry or in some other way unsettled by reflecting on clinical work.

Other blocks to receiving clinical supervision

As well as the difficulties that may arise in engaging in supervision from the personal perspective, there are also a number of very persuasive reasons for not getting supervision that may operate on a more conscious level of understanding that take into account not only the personal, but also the organisational difficulties that the supervisee may face when setting out to establish a supervision relationship. These can include:

PREVIOUS EXPERIENCE

A person's previous experience of supervision whether this has been good or bad may be the stumbling block that prevents them from being supervised in the future. What they remember of previous supervision may result in the supervisee not wishing to relive a previous poor experience, or feeling that no other supervisor could possibly match the excellence of the last one.

ORGANISATIONAL INTERFERENCE
This may take a number of forms including a confusion between
managerial supervision and supervision on the part of senior
nurse managers. This can result in the supervisee feeling
unsupported in terms of the time and appropriate personnel
being made available.

LACK OF SKILLS
This may or may not be connected to the organisational blocks
mentioned above. The supervisee finds it difficult to locate
suitably qualified and skilled clinical supervisors within his
locality, perhaps due to financial or geographical difficulties.

CULTURAL BLOCKS
Cultural blocks result in a difficulty in receiving the feedback.
They can be a consequence of language barriers or more personal
reasons. It may, for example, feel safer for the supervisee to be a
provider of care than a receiver of it.

**Think about . . . professional and organisational blocks to clinical
supervision**

Read the list of possible 'blocks' to supervision that nurses may encounter
and then address the following questions.

1 How many of them relate to your own experiences of receiving or
   considering supervision?
2 Are there any other 'stumbling blocks' that you have encountered
   either in yourself or in others that are not listed?
3 Imagine chatting with a nurse who is experiencing a block towards
   supervision in each of the areas listed above. How would you start to
   address their concerns in order that they feel less threatened and
   more inclined to accept clinical supervision?

2
What is the Point of Clinical Supervision?

Key issues in this chapter

- Where and why clinical supervision began
- Supervision in health visiting, mental health nursing and midwifery
- Three descriptions of clinical supervision
- The functions of clinical supervision
- The link between nurse mentoring and clinical supervision

A brief history of clinical supervision: where it all began

Burns (1958) has shown that clinical nursing supervision – in its current form – probably began to be practised seriously, regularly and by a significant number of people in the early 1920s. It grew out of the theories and practice of psychoanalysis, and it has become a mandatory feature for practitioners in this field, existing as a source of professional enhancement, education and support. Clinical supervision for psychoanalysists, psychotherapists and psychodynamic counsellors often operates on a weekly basis and many professional associations require practitioners to maintain regular – and relevant – supervision for their work, sometimes at their own cost and in their own time. A usual minimum requirement is weekly supervision for each style of therapy being practised (including individual, group and family therapies). Consequently, it is not uncommon for therapists and counsellors to attend more than one clinical supervision session each week.

Children's nurses, health visitors, mental health nurses and midwives

Within nursing, midwifery and health visiting, certain specialist branches of the profession have been advocating and – to some extent – practising clinical supervision for many decades. Bond and Holland (1998) have identified health visitors, children's nurses, midwives and mental health nurses amongst those nursing and nursing-related groups that have particularly embraced the concept of clinical supervision as an integral part of their professional activity.

Health visitors and children's nurses – spare the rod and supervise the nurses

It is apparent, from the work of Bond and Holland, that a supervisory structure for health visitors and children's nurses is well-established. The problem seems to be that it has at its core the extremely important – but to my mind, narrowly focused – primary aim of protecting the patients but with less emphasis on the education and support of the practitioners themselves. The protection of vulnerable children is not at issue here, and I hope that my view of its crucial importance will not be doubted. What I am prepared to dispute is the validity of the general structure and philosophy of any supervisory system that concerns itself only with one aspect of a process that holds so much potential for professionals and patients alike.

Mental health nurses – Sigmund Who?

The legacy that psychotherapy has bequeathed to its 'kissing-cousin' mental health nursing is, perhaps, an unquestioning acceptance of the recognised principles and advantages of clinical supervision. Unfortunately, it would seem that although mental health nurses might appear to have embraced the concepts of clinical supervision, there is not always an obvious willingness to put them into practice. A number of writers have suggested that the practice of clinical supervision by mental health nurses is still only being carried out in a limited and piecemeal fashion. From my own experience, clinical supervision has long been an important focus of mental health nurses working in more specialist fields including community mental health nursing and nurses specialising in the practice of psychodynamic, behavioural and cognitive-behavioural therapies. Faugier (1996) supports the view that community mental health nurses have traditionally had better established systems of clinical supervision than those based at in-patient units.

The increasing trend in some mental health nursing organisations, of commitment to training nurses in supervision skills and the formulation of policies designed to ensure that all mental health nurses receive a minimum amount of clinical supervision each year, has, fortunately, begun to redress the balance in favour of those mental health nurses working in in-patient settings.

Midwives – an inspector calls

According to Bond and Holland (1998: 27), midwives have been supervised since 1936, when the title of 'Inspector of Midwives' was changed to that of 'Supervisor of Midwives'. The model of supervision generally adopted by midwives appears however, to be a standards-based one which, according to Bent (1992) is directed by the guiding principle that the safety of mother and baby is at 'the very heart of supervision'. There is a strong link, here, between the supervisory process and the disciplinary procedure and Bond and Holland contend that important supervisory elements such as support and professional growth are not always obvious within the structure of midwifery supervision, despite what they describe as hopeful statements to the contrary. Bent points to an early signpost for the appropriate direction of midwifery supervision in a document from a departmental committee of 1929 which wisely advises that: 'an inspector of midwives should be regarded as the counsellor and friend of the midwives rather than a relentless critic . . . and make them feel that there is always someone to whom they can look for sympathetic understanding' (Bent, 1992: 7).

What IS clinical supervision?

Philip Bromberg (1982) posed a salient question that should, in my view, be asked by – and of – all those engaged in the task of clinical nursing supervision: 'What goes on in this two-person field called supervision that makes it succeed in its aim? What is it I am doing when I supervise and what is it I think I am doing?' (1982: 193).

I think of clinical supervision as a potentially safe environment in which practitioners can gain fresh insights, discuss new ideas and develop self-awareness (Power, 1994a). The supervisory process, at its best, allows for an objective overview of the therapist–patient relationship, within the relative security of a safe environment, in which the supervisee can be offered a unique opportunity to explore the often complicated dynamics of their professional yet personal relationship with their patients.

Three descriptions of clinical supervision

There are numerous and varied descriptions of clinical supervision to be found in the existing literature. As far as nursing is concerned, there are several examples of workable descriptions of supervision to choose from and three particularly pragmatic ones are offered here. The first description originates from The Community Psychiatric Nurses' Association and perhaps uses language that might seem more familiar to those nurses working in specialised areas of therapy or counselling but is no less relevant to nurses working in other fields. The second definition is from Target 10 in the Department of Health's 1993 strategy paper for nursing and health visiting – 'A vision for the future'. For the third definition I have combined key statement 1 and key statement 2 from the UKCC's *Position Statement On Clinical Supervision* (1996).

1   Clinical nursing supervision is . . .

> . . . A dynamic, interpersonally focused experience which promotes the development of therapeutic proficiency. One of the primary reasons for all supervision is that the quality of therapeutic work with the client is of a consistently high standard in relation to the client's needs. Consequently supervision must be acknowledged as a corner-stone of clinical practice. (Community Psychiatric Nurses' Association (CPNA), 1989)

2   Clinical nursing supervision is . . .

> . . . the term used to describe a formal process of professional support and learning which enables practitioners to develop knowledge and competence, assume responsibility for their own practice and enhance consumer protection and the safety of care in complex clinical situations. It is central to the process of learning and to the expansion of the scope of practice and should be seen as the means for encouraging self-assessment and analytic and reflective skills. (Department of Health, 1993)

3   Clinical nursing supervision is . . .

. . . a practice-focused professional relationship involving a practitioner reflecting on practice guided by a skilled supervisor. [It] supports practice, enabling practitioners to maintain and promote standards of care. (United Kingdom Central Council for Nursing and Midwifery (UKCC), 1996)

Think about . . . the common denominators of clinical supervision

After you have read each of the descriptions, above, take a few minutes to think about them and then address the following questions, before moving on.

1   What do these definitions of clinical nursing supervision have in common?
2   Can you find key words that suggest common themes linking two or all three of the descriptions together?

In my view, some similarities in the descriptions of clinical nursing supervision include:

- Reflection on clinical practice, leading to its enhancement.
- Promotion of professional standards and quality of care.
- Skills (of: practice, reflection, analysis and supervision).

There are other aspects of supervision that are also worthy of consideration. My suggestions for some other important elements of clinical supervision are:

- The patient's needs and their protection.
- The process of learning by the supervisee.
- The professional support of the supervisee.
- The safety of the supervisee's nursing practice.
- The supervisee's sense of responsibility for his own nursing practice.
- The capacity of the supervisee to monitor and assess his nursing practice.

By combining some of the important aspects outlined so far, I will offer a six-point plan for the purpose and direction of clinical nursing supervision in nursing.

al supervision in nursing should . . .

flect upon the supervisee's nursing practice.
2   Promote learning and advancement of skills.
3   Be skills-based in its application.
4   Be supportive of the supervisee and open to changing needs.
5   Have the best interests of the patient as the highest priority.
6   Encourage safe and independent practice.

A pragmatic proposition for clinical supervision
A model of supervision described originally by Kadushin (1992) and intended for social workers, suggests that the primary components of clinical supervision should be:

● Education
● Support
● Management

Proctor (1986), examining the functions of clinical supervision specifically from a nursing standpoint, also separates the primary components of clinical supervision into three major categories. Although her categories have similar intentions to those described by Kadushin, Proctor uses radically different terms to describe their aims in a way that she feels is more in keeping with the practice of nursing. Proctor's three primary components of clinical supervision are:

● *Formative* – focusing on issues of education and professional development for the supervisee.
● *Restorative* – focusing on issues of support with an aim of avoiding 'burn-out' and loss of morale in the supervisee.
● *Normative* – focusing on issues of personal organisation, ethics and quality in the nursing care practised by the supervisee.

I will now offer a six-point pragmatic proposal for the purpose and direction of clinical supervision in nursing by integrating the principles of clinical supervision for nurses outlined in the descriptions above, with my aims cited above and incorporating the arguments examining the three primary functions, as described by both Kadushin (1992) and Proctor (1986).

The objectives of clinical supervision

Supervision should reflect upon the supervisee's nursing practice

Nursing practice is dependent upon, and should be guided by, nursing knowledge. Unfortunately, these two integral strands of the profession, nursing-theory and nursing-practice, have often failed to 'gel' together in a way that satisfies both the nurse educationalists and the nurse practitioners equally. As a consequence, the so-called 'theory–practice gap' is still very much alive and well and living in the heart of many nursing organisations. Reed and Procter (1993) feel that an issue that needs to be addressed in nursing is not only *what* particular knowledge should be applied to the practice of nursing, but also just *how* that knowledge should be properly disseminated throughout the profession. They state that practice should be concerned with intervention and that knowledge and action are brought together, presumably to the ultimate benefit of the patient. Schön (1987) was also concerned that practitioners should be able to: 'select judiciously from the myriad theoretical perspectives they have learnt, those that are appropriate to the particular case with which they are confronted' (Reed and Procter, 1993: 25).

Because patients often present nurses with what Reed and Procter describe as 'specific and sometimes contradictory problems', safe nursing practice demands that the nurse adopts a process of procedure selection that cannot be wholly based on rational academic knowledge, but one that is based on a combination of theory and the experience gained through the actual practice of nursing. Reed and Procter, with reference to Schön state that 'This practice-based knowledge . . . is a characteristic of the way in which professionals know about their world, a way in which he called *reflective practice*' (1993: 25, emphasis added).

Reflective practice should, ideally, be a balanced combination of the theoretical and the pragmatic. It should also involve a constant review of the action taken with patients whilst considering the available knowledge-base in direct relation to the practical nursing situation faced. Clinical supervision can offer the ideal forum for such a review of knowledge and practice.

WHAT NURSES SHOULD TALK ABOUT DURING CLINICAL SUPERVISION

Hawkins and Shohet (1989) have described four main elements involved in clinical supervision: the supervisor, the supervisee, the client and a work context. I have adapted this model, originally designed for a more generic readership, to put a greater emphasis on clinical supervision in nursing and my own preference for a broader term than client. Therefore, I would suggest that the four elements present in any clinical nursing supervision session are:

1   The supervisor
2   The supervisee
3   The patient
4   A nursing context

These four elements will always be present, either in a real and tangible way, or in some other way – usually through talking, thinking and feeling about them – as with the patient and the work context. The supervisor has a role to play in guiding the supervisee toward thinking about the patient and helping to maintain a connection between the supervisee, the patient and the working environment, the clinical situation and the task of nursing in general. Although it may seem superfluous to suggest that clinical nursing supervision should be about the practice of nursing, I feel that it does bear stating, and re-stating, in order that its use becomes as seriously considered and respected as any other clinical aspect of nursing.

One of the most tempting things, for me at least, about having someone who is prepared to give some of their time to listen and talk is to say whatever comes into my head. The weather; the TV drama I watched last night; my changing physical appearance; my application for another nursing post all spring to mind as potential fodder to fire at the unsuspecting supportive listener. But which topics would my supervisor want to have me talk about?

The short answer is: any topic that has a direct connection to my clinical nursing work. Some topics may be more obvious than others and present themselves more readily to the supervisee. Talking about a television drama to my clinical supervisor might seem like a pointless and time-wasting exercise, but what if it featured a character that reminded me of a client that I am working with, and had triggered off several new ideas about my work with that person? It might suddenly become relevant and a new source of information to assist the supervisory process.

Many nurses new to receiving clinical nursing supervision, may not feel safe about talking to someone who does not have more experience than themselves in their specific aspect of nursing. Some supervisors may also have qualms about offering supervision to someone that they suspect may be more skilled or experienced than they are in certain aspects of the work. I suggest that as much consideration as possible should be given to the question of how the supervisee can be helped to have initial – and increasing – confidence in his supervisor. That said, I believe that it is perfectly possible for the supervisor to achieve the aim of appropriately focusing on the clinical work of the supervisee, without being or becoming an 'expert' in it herself.

Clinical supervision should promote learning and advancement of skills

The educational (or formative) element of clinical supervision is concerned with developing the skills, understanding and abilities of the supervisee. This is achieved through encouraging the supervisee to reflect on the nursing care being practised, together with guided exploration of the supervisee's assessment, implementation and evaluation of his work with the patients. Some of the aims of this aspect of clinical supervision include:

- Understanding the supervisee's clinical situation as fully as possible.
- Helping the supervisee become aware of their reactions and responses to the patients.
- Exploring the dynamics of their interactions with patients.
- Examining how the supervisee acted with patients and the consequences of those actions.

Clinical supervision should be skills-based in its application

There are several practical ways in which supervisors may achieve the aims of the educational component of supervision.

- Through examination of the case material presented.
- By focusing on the supervisee's direct interventions.
- By encouraging an awareness of the dynamics occurring between the supervisee and the patient.
- By helping the supervisee to explore other ways of working than the methods currently being presented to the supervisor.

Bromberg (1982) sees himself as an 'educator' when he supervises other clinicians and uses the term to describe someone who participates in the supervisory relationship, with the intention of facilitating the supervisee's capacity to function more effectively. If the educational component of clinical supervision was similar to that of teaching someone how to operate a piece of machinery then it would, states Bromberg, be a relatively simple matter of transmitting a body of knowledge from the supervisor to the supervisee, while the task was being performed. However, the process of supervision is different from giving instructions to a machine operator in that there is a living person with a mind of their own (the patient) at the 'core' of the teaching. This has an important bearing on the instruction given because the patient's own actions may conflict with, confuse or even totally negate the conclusions drawn during clinical supervision.

Klauber (1980) likened the process of education in clinical supervision to that of teaching someone to play a card game. In this analogy, the third party involved (the card player's opponent) is also a living person, with a mind of her own, who may make unpredicted moves. Klauber argues that the essential ingredient necessary for the 'card-player' (the supervisee) to learn, and which is not required when learning to use machinery, is spontaneity. This is relevant, I suggest, because nurses frequently have to 'think on their feet' – and respond spontaneously – when their patients show a 'hand of cards' that the nurse did not expect them to 'play'.

Clinical supervision should be supportive of the supervisee and open to changing needs

The second major component of clinical supervision is the supportive (or restorative) one. This strand of clinical supervision is concerned with the way the supervisee responds to the demands of nursing. The emotional distress that many nurses experience is due – in part – to the very necessary empathy required by the dynamics of the relationship (Faugier, 1996). If nurses are to maintain control of their personal feelings as they go about their day-to-day activities, as well as a feeling of stability and the ability to construct and maintain professional boundaries, it is essential that they become aware of how the work has affected them personally, in order that they can appropriately deal with their emotional reactions to it.

Hawkins and Shohet (1989) relate this aspect of supervision to the British coal miners of the 1920s, who won the right to wash off the grime of the job in the pit-owner's time, rather than having to go home to their families still dirty from the day's toils, and wash it off there, if they could. The supportive (or restorative) element in supervision is the emotional and some would argue, therapeutic equivalent of the miner's 'pithead time'. The nurse who is appropriately exposed to this aspect of supervision learns to leave the 'grime' at work and – hopefully – goes home carrying less distress, dis-ease and fragmentation of spirit and personality.

The main aims of the supportive/restorative component of supervision include:

- Preventing the supervisee from becoming overburdened with emotions about the patients.
- Helping the supervisee to understand the origins of these emotions.
- Assisting the supervisee to build and maintain professional boundaries.
- Encouraging the supervisee to avoid over-identification with the patients, which may in itself lead to problems in delivering nursing care.
- Assisting the prevention of professional 'burn-out'.

One note of caution in relation to this component of clinical supervision is sounded by McNeill and Worthen (1989). They argue that some supervisors may be reluctant to discuss personal issues in the supervision session for fear of placing themselves in an ethical dilemma concerning the dual role as both supervisor and personal therapist for a supervisee. They stress that supervision should not become therapy as this would result in a confusing and unhelpful situation for the supervisee.

Supervision should have the best interests of the patient as its highest priority

The managerial (or normative) aspect of supervision is, according to Faugier (1996), 'the crucial quality-control element' and it is important because:

> Even the most experienced . . . nurse will have inevitable blind-spots, human failings, areas of vulnerability and woundedness from her internal and external world and prejudices of which she may remain blithely unaware. This aspect of the model emphasises that when someone becomes a supervisor, he/she is duty-bound to ensure that the highest professional standards . . . are upheld and that the policies and procedures of the authority are followed. (Faugier, 1996)

Think about . . . blind spots and failings

Implicit in the quote above from Faugier (1996), is the suggestion that there are factors in the nursing relationship that may be:

- Ignored or overlooked by the nurse.
- Outside the control of the nurse.
- Open to a potentially negative response from the nurse.

1 How common do you feel such occurrences are in nursing?
2 Can you recall situations where a colleague has:
   a) expressed negative opinions of patients?
   b) avoided nursing certain patients?
   c) negatively over-reacted to the 'demands' of some patients?
3 How likely is it that colleagues could point out similar situations concerning yourself?
4 How could clinical supervision help to redress such situations?

Nurses – often despite our own attempts to have the rest of the world believe otherwise – are subject to all the usual human frailties and failings. We have blind spots, prejudices and vulnerabilities just as others do – even when we are at work, caring for others. We have the capacity to become ignorant, of people we would rather not have contact with; requests we would prefer not to carry out; failings in ourselves and others we choose not to recognise; and of rules and regulations, if we believe that 'bending' them may be of benefit to ourselves or others. We can forget to do certain unpleasant tasks and take longer over the more enjoyable parts of our work. We can easily do the wrong thing at the right time and the right thing at the wrong time. We can choose who we would prefer to nurse and who we would prefer to leave well alone. We can offer preferential treatment to some lucky souls and the cold shoulder to the not-so-lucky.

We can do all of these things – and more – because we are human. These human traits – even though we may sometimes wish that they did not exist – do have the potential to interfere with and detract from our capacity to offer the highest possible standards of nursing care.

Sometimes we can do these things deliberately and with full awareness of our actions and the probable consequences of them, but more often than not, we do them without fully understanding how, why, or even if what we are doing is detrimental, harmful, inconsiderate or in some other way not in the best interests of some of the people we are charged with nursing.

Clinical nursing supervision is conducted for the nurse – the provider of nursing care – but it is ultimately and fundamentally concerned with those on the receiving end of nursing care. It is the patients who should be the first priority for consideration by the supervisor and supervisee, during the clinical supervision session.

Clinical supervision should encourage safe practice

Nurse managers and nursing organisation executives regularly refer to the almost magical, and sometimes elusive notion, of the 'value-added' ingredient that clinical supervision can provide. It is probably fair to say that, for those nurses in the position of managing large budgets and needing to justify additional expenditure – in terms of both time and money – a decision to implement clinical supervision within an area of the nursing organisation will often be made in relation to the perceived increase in 'value', or enhanced professionalism, that it brings to the existing service. Not only will the best interests of the patients be served from the increase in skills and knowledge and sense of supported practice inherent in regular, competent supervision, but nurses will also gain an enhanced sense of themselves as safe and independent practitioners.

What is NOT the point of clinical supervision?

If clinical nursing supervision is to work it should not be allowed to become:

- A management activity allowing for the over-seeing of subordinates.
- Linked to the disciplinary process.
- Exclusively concerned with time-keeping, rates of pay, hours of duty, and rostering.
- About having the supervisee's work controlled, directed or managerially evaluated.
- A punitive or gratuitously negative experience for the supervisee.
- A continuous discussion of mistakes, failings or errors on the part of the supervisee, without being balanced by a discussion of the supervisee's professional strengths and the positive aspects of his work.

A brief survey of the nursing literature (including Platt-Koch, 1986) suggests, however, that for many nurses, clinical nursing supervision is all of those negative, restrictive and discouraging things in the above – and will remain so – until outmoded attitudes and ways of functioning in nursing environments change dramatically. In order to ensure that clinical nursing supervision is regarded positively by an increasing number of nurses in all areas of the work, there needs to be a common understanding of its true and intended purpose and as a consequence, clear structures within the nursing environment to avoid confusion and conflict.

The mentoring–clinical supervision connection

The concept of clinical supervision for nurses is frequently connected to, and perhaps also frequently confused with, other similar roles within nursing such as that of the nurse-mentor. I firmly believe that mentoring should be regarded as a separate nursing role, and one that is best understood when associated with the task of facilitating the change from one nursing role or position to another. Mentors, in the true nursing sense, are usually involved in guiding and assisting another nurse through a transitional period of change – perhaps from 'newly qualified novice' to 'competent practitioner' (as with preceptorship) or from 'experienced clinical practitioner' to competent nurse-lecturer or nurse-manager. That said, and putting the assessment (or grading) component of the nurse-mentor role aside, there is much in common with the role and desired-characteristics of the clinical nurse supervisor.

The classical origins of mentoring

East (1995) explains how mentoring has its origins in Greek mythology. The Greek poet, Homer tells the story of Odysseus, King of Ithaca, who while away fighting in the Trojan War, entrusted his young son, Telemachus, to the care of a guardian – named Mentor. Odysseus was prevented from returning home for ten years, and the Goddess Athena – the daughter of Zeus but who was neither all-powerful nor all-wise – was moved by his plight. Athena, who is often connected with war, but who was also patroness of Arts and Crafts, occasionally the Goddess of Medicine, and ultimately, the Goddess of Wisdom, assumed the appearance of Mentor, to make an earthly visit and assist the young and inexperienced Telemachus in making a rescue bid for his father. Thereafter, Athena would appear to Telemachus as Mentor whenever she wanted to offer him advice and guidance in his attempt to save his father. Athena combined her practical skills with insight and wisdom and a capacity to support and guide others in their attempt to achieve the highest goals and took on many different roles in order to achieve this.

As with the concept of clinical supervision, there is a wide range of definitions concerning the role of the mentor, both generally and within nursing specifically. Levinson (1978), cited in East (1995), states that the mentor is someone who, whether employed in nursing or elsewhere, should: 'facilitate life transitions . . . by allowing the mentee to be a novice or apprentice to a more advanced expert and authoritative adult' (1995: 111). East adds that the origins of mentoring are to be found in the concepts of apprenticeship. In his view, the mentor becomes involved in a relationship which is initiated, often formally, by an organisation in order to achieve results similar to those of the classical relationship, as part of a structured staff development programme.

In addition to the notion of apprenticeship, there are many connections with 'guidance' associated with mentoring. Rowntree describes the mentor as: 'a trusted and friendly advisor or guide, especially of someone new to a particular role' (1981: 64) and Daloz underscores the concept of the mentor as a 'guide' with his view that: 'The mentor should act as a travelling companion – who is a more trusted guide than a "tour director"' (1986: 29).

East (1995) suggests that the first reference to mentors in nursing, and as part of course approval processes, was made in the ENB circular (1987/28/MAT) which defines a mentor as: 'an appropriately qualified and experienced first level nurse who, by example and facilitation, guides assists and supports the student in learning new skills, adopting new behaviours and acquiring new attitudes' (1995: 119). East supports and complements these descriptions with her own view that: 'the mentor represents knowledge, reflection, insight, understanding, good advice, determination and planning. Qualities which cannot be mastered alone' (1995: 120). East argues however, that the mentoring role in nursing is often restricted to offering support for tasks linked to achieving professional and vocational qualifications and that this component should be more correctly defined as 'pseudo' or 'quasi-mentoring' because the focus of the mentee is mainly on gaining professional qualifications. East feels that the definition of true mentoring should be reserved for those situations in which one nurse offers 'holistic support' for another nurse in the development of a new and complex professional role.

I was appointed to my first nurse-lecturer post, after more than twenty years as a clinically-based mental health nurse, with some standing and several years experience as a clinical supervisor. It was, strangely enough, the first time in my career that I had ever been allocated a 'mentor' in the generally accepted nursing sense. The prospect was quite daunting. There was I, an experienced and highly qualified nurse, being subjected to scrutiny, guidance, advice and – worst of all – assessment for almost two years during my education training period, from someone with perhaps less clinical experience than me. Should I be offended? Would I be de-skilled? Would I be difficult and rebel? Was there a good reason why someone with my experience should require a mentor? Had I been asked these questions at the beginning of my mentoring period, I would have answered with an unerring 'yes' to the first three and an emphatic 'no' to the fourth. Had I been asked them just a few weeks into my mentoring period, the answers would have been reversed. My mentor became an important guide, teacher, role-model and assessor on my 'journey of transition', as I now see it, from experienced clinical nurse to inexperienced nurse-lecturer and beyond. Without his support and encouragement, I would have made many more mistakes and it would have undoubtedly taken me much longer to achieve a state of 'independent competence' as a nurse-lecturer.

3

The Question(s) of Clinical Supervision

Key issues in this chapter

- Packing for the journey to clinical supervision
- Negative capability
- Becoming a clinical nurse supervisor
- The right setting for clinical supervision
- The qualities required of a clinical nurse supervisor
- The legal considerations of clinical supervision

So many questions, so few right answers

There are so many questions asked about clinical supervision that it can sometimes seem surprising that its practice ever begins at all. The disappointing truth is that, in some nursing organisations, it never does start. Some nurses get 'stuck' in the state of asking *all* of the questions and needing to know *all* of the answers before feeling safe about setting off on the journey into the uncharted territory of clinical supervision – which, of course, they never do!

Pack your own bag

But no sensible traveller ever sets off totally unprepared for a journey. She packs a bag with the essential items for survival and perhaps, a few luxuries. However, if a hundred different travellers were to be asked exactly what they pack for any given journey, the result might be a hundred different lists. We all consider different things to be important. An item that one person cannot possibly live without may not even be in the bag of her travelling companion. Starting off down the road of clinical supervision is similar, in that we will have a list of essential items that we need to put in our psychological bag before we feel ready to set off. The choices we make in terms of which questions to ask and which answers we require will often be as personal and idiosyncratic as packing a bag for a journey.

Stop the trip, I forgot my toothbrush!

Imagine a holiday-maker, listening to cabin crew explain the use of the emergency equipment as the plane moves down the runway for take-off. Suddenly, she remembers that she forgot to pack what she considers to be an important item of luggage. Does she shout 'stop the 'plane and let me off!' Does she arrive at her holiday resort but return home immediately? I doubt it. I think that the sensible traveller might consider just how important that missing item is to the successful completion of the journey. Can she live without it? Can she obtain something similar during her trip? Is it worth cancelling the entire trip for the sake of something that she can probably live without or obtain later? Does she, perhaps, think carefully about what she already has in her bag and wonder if those items are enough at least to be going on with. Does she decide that she has enough luggage to enjoy the trip in the knowledge that it is likely to bring about new insights and new horizons?

For me, the journey into clinical supervision for nurses is not that different from any other trip into a new place. My advice to new travellers is to pack your own bag with those items that you already possess which you consider essential. Try to enjoy the journey, bearing in mind that anything you don't possess can most likely be gathered along the way, should you feel you need it.

But before setting off, consider the only item that I consider as a *must* for anyone considering a trip into new psychological territory and the one that, to some extent, turns all the items from 'essentials' to 'luxuries' – *negative capability*.

Be positive – try negative capability!

The poet, John Keats, coined the phrase *negative capability* in a letter to his brothers in 1817. He described the phenomenon as the psychological capacity of: '. . . being in uncertainties, mysteries, doubts, without any irritable reaching after fact and reason' (Keats, 1817, in Casement, 1985: 223).

The need to *know* is a fundamental human trait. Media empires have been built around our need to be kept informed; novelists have made fortunes from slowly unfolding the identity of the serial axe-murderer and song-writers seem to frequently express the pain of waiting to hear who their ex-lover is 'holding-in-his/ her-arms-tonight', in e-minor.

The psychoanalyst Wilfred Bion (1980), did not believe that the need to know everything about a given situation should be of paramount concern for practitioners. Rather than advocating any comfort from *knowing*, he was very concerned about maintaining a positive attitude towards the idea of *not-knowing* everything all at once. Bion argued that:

> Instead of trying to bring a brilliant, intelligent, knowledgeable light to bear on obscure problems . . . we bring to bear a diminuation of the 'light' – a penetrating beam of darkness; a reciprocal of the searchlight . . . The darkness would be so absolute that it would achieve a luminous, absolute vacuum . . . if any object existed, however faint, it would show up very clearly. (Bion, 1974, in Casement, 1985: 222–3)

Over forty-five years earlier, Sigmund Freud, the so-called father of psychoanalysis expressed his views on the problems of dogmatic opinion and too firmly fixed beliefs and ideas caused by human beings 'creating a store of ideas . . . born from man's need to make his helplessness tolerable' (Freud, 1927: 18). Freud was possibly suggesting that in order to make ourselves feel safe as human beings – when in fact we are potentially very vulnerable and fragile – we have amassed a great deal of information and beliefs that we can call on when we are feeling particularly threatened, as a sort of psychological comfort blanket.

The need to know applies to nurses and potential clinical supervision participants as much as anyone else. I am not advocating that, as nurses, we do nothing to enhance our knowledge and skills – that is, after all, one of the main advantages of clinical supervision – but I am suggesting that it is possible to start a new venture without knowing all about it and everything that is involved.

Many years ago, an experienced supervisor listened patiently to my concerns arising from my attempts to study psychotherapy:

> *Me*: . . . I read all the time – long into the night studying all the books I can get my hands on, memorising various models and theories of psychotherapy; I watch videos about expert therapists displaying their skills; I attend conferences and listen attentively while renowned speakers contradict the experts in the books that I have

read and watch experts display different skills that work just as well as the ones on the videos. At the end of the day, I am left feeling confused and somewhat inadequate. It's as if all I have learnt from my endeavours, so far, is how much I have still yet to learn!
Supervisor: That sounds like progress.

To know some of the *questions* you need to ask can be as important as knowing the answers. So read on, pack your psychological bag as well as you feel able, and when you know for sure that you still do not – and will never – know *everything*, you will at last know that you are making some progress.

Some frequently asked questions of clinical supervision

In this section I will address some of the questions about clinical supervision that have been important to myself and many of the supervisees and supervisors that I have encountered on my own journey. I hope that they will prove helpful for others too, but do try to remember the essential item of *negative capability*, which should help you to at least embark on this interesting and potentially very fruitful journey no matter what else may (or may not) be in your bag as you set off.

Who should become a clinical supervisor?
The question 'who should supervise nurses?' is perhaps almost as impossible to answer simply and succinctly as: 'how long should a piece of naso-gastric tubing be?' Rather, it is probably simpler, and more useful, to think about who should *not* be chosen as a clinical supervisor. I will begin to answer this question, then, with a short-list of the type of nurses that first-time supervisees should consider *avoiding* as their clinical supervisor.

A BASIC RULE-OF-THUMB FOR CHOOSING YOUR FIRST CLINICAL SUPERVISOR

- No nurse to whom you are managerially accountable or responsible.
- No nurse who has never had experience in your area of clinical practice.
- No nurse who is less qualified and/or experienced than yourself.
- No nurse who has very limited experience of and/or no formal training in clinical supervision.

The above list can be used as a rough guide by nurses seeking supervision for the first time. It may not be relevant to all nurses looking for clinical supervision but a supervision priority should be to ensure that the first experience is perceived as positive, safe and one that encourages the supervisee to continue. The more precautions we take to ensure supervisees experience these things, the more likely they are to return to supervision on a regular basis. In addition to the above short-list, there are also certain conditions that I feel should be adhered to whenever a nurse chooses to embark on clinical supervision.

- The supervisee should choose to be in supervision.
- The supervisee should not be managerially responsible to the supervisor.
- The supervisee should not be required to attend supervision for any managerial or disciplinary reason.
- The supervisee should feel that he can stop attending clinical supervision without being punished or penalised.

How do nurses become clinical supervisors?
Becoming a clinical supervisor is a step that a nurse should take carefully and with considerable thought to:

- Her reasons for choosing to become a clinical nurse supervisor.
- The particular qualities that she brings to the process.
- The preparation that she may need in order to supervise safely and effectively.

Why do nurses become clinical supervisors?
Nurses may choose to become clinical supervisors for a variety of reasons; some obviously connected to the professional and organisational responsibilities that they have and others more to do with their own personal wishes and needs. Whether the decision to clinically supervise other nurses is based on tangible, professional requirements and organisational directives or more personal issues and concerns, it is essential that the prospective supervisor considers her motives carefully.

It would be professionally unsound, in my view, for a senior nurse to undertake the role of clinical supervisor, purely on the grounds that the organisational structure is moving towards clinical supervision for all staff, and the obvious choice for supervisors are the most senior nurses in the team.

The potential supervisor should think long and hard about her motives for wanting to adopt this role. After all, it carries no managerial authority; probably will not – in itself – warrant a salary increase; is likely to involve an increased workload and work-rate and a lot of people will find it hard to understand just *why* she has chosen to go to the trouble of burdening herself with the problems of one or more colleagues, when surely she has enough of her own to contend with, doesn't she?

The box below contains some of the things that you should confront yourself with as a first stage in sorting the supervisory wheat from the chaff. Use it as a semi-serious (and reasonably transparent) test that should, if nothing else, give you some food for thought about your motives for choosing clinical supervision as an extension of your role.

Think about . . . wanting to become a clinical supervisor

Quickly answer YES or NO to each of the questions, then check your scores below and use the questions (and your score) as food for thought about the validity of your decision to become a clinical supervisor.

1 Will you gain, professionally or personally from supervising other nurses?
2 Do you feel that clinical supervision is glamorous or status-enhancing?
3 Is it important that senior nurses become clinical supervisors in order to extend their managerial role?
4 Should the clinical supervisor's views be open to question or disagreement by the supervisee?
5 Is clinical supervision nothing more than a new-fangled way of controlling junior nurses?
6 As clinical supervisor are you obliged to teach the supervisee everything you know?
7 Is it important that nurses are challenged, probed and generally prompted to think about their work on a regular basis?
8 Would your position within the nursing team be undermined if you chose not to become a clinical supervisor?

Scoring:
Q1: YES=2 NO=0, **Q2**: YES=2 NO=0, **Q3**: YES=2 NO=0,
Q4: YES=0 NO=2 **Q5**: YES=2 NO=0, **Q6**: YES=2 NO=0,
Q7: YES=0 NO=2, **Q8**: YES=2 NO=0

The verdict:
0–2 points: You are probably very well suited to considering clinical supervision and/or you worked out the scoring system.
2–8 points: There are some good reasons to become a clinical supervisor and you may be discovering them – keep thinking about them.
10–16 points: Either you are probably more suited to managerial supervision or you have been playing games with yourself on this test. Whatever the reason for your high score, I suggest that you have a rethink about whether or not you are considering clinical supervision for the right reasons!

What are the essential characteristics for clinical supervisors?

The essential characteristics for clinical supervisors discussed here are to a large extent based on the work of Jean Faugier (1992, 1996) and encompass a range of human qualities that the supervisor will demonstrate during the supervision sessions. Faugier has outlined a range of supervisor characteristics that are often evident in positive and successful clinical supervision for nurses and are key elements of her 'growth and support model' of clinical supervision. Faugier advocates the role of supervisor as a facilitator of growth in the supervisee and a provider of the essential requirement of support, which allows the supervisee to move safely towards the practice of clinical excellence. I will use Faugier's growth and support model to outline some of the key elements and characteristics that I feel are important and desirable in clinical supervisors of nurses.

GENEROSITY

Faugier regards generosity as an essential requirement for supervisors, who need to be generous with their *time* – acknowledging that supervision takes precedence over all other activities – barring emergencies; and their *spirit*, by giving to the supervisee intellectually and emotionally.

REWARDING

The supervisor needs to be able to recognise and reward ability. Faugier states that a prerequisite to the 'rewarding' characteristic in a clinical supervisor is *self-awareness*. The more a person is 'comfortable' with herself, the more she will be able to offer praise and inspiration, when appropriate.

OPENNESS
The supervisor must be open to the notion that a potentially very wide range of emotional and physiological issues can be presented, daily, to supervisees by patients. This can lead to difficulties within the supervisory relationship itself for which the supervisor must be prepared, and able, to deal with objectively and professionally.

WILLINGNESS TO LEARN
The ability of supervisors to continue to learn throughout their careers is an important element of the growth and support model. The consequence of not continuing along the path of career-long learning is that supervisors are in danger of being 'engulfed by the oncoming tide of development represented by the person of their supervisees' (Faugier, 1996: 61).

THOUGHTFUL AND THOUGHT-PROVOKING
The Support and Growth model sees the supervisor as a proactive being who wishes to provide the right environment for supervision while simultaneously demonstrating competence as a senior clinical nurse. When this condition is allied to the needs of the supervisee, who wishes to increase his knowledge and skills and the needs of the nursing organisation, who wish to ensure that the patients are given the highest standards of care, the supervisor will be required to demonstrate a capacity for thoughtful and thought-provoking action.

HUMANITY
Humanity is a condition that needs to be present in order for the supervision to be conducted in a way that reflects the nurse's capacity to treat the patients as valued human beings, and not just the objects of professional attention. I also feel that that humanity is a quality required in the supervisor in order that it can be maintained, and even germinated and grown, in her supervisee.

SENSITIVITY
The supervisor must be sensitive to the struggles and frustrations that supervisees endure in practice, and discuss in supervision. It is important for the supervisor to respond to her supervisee in a way that acknowledges the level of work expended and any sense of failure and guilt that may surround her supervisee's concern that he has failed to achieve as much as was hoped for. If the

supervisor demonstrates sufficient level of sensitivity it will be less likely that her supervisee will try to cover up mistakes and concerns with silence and avoidance of the problem.

UNCOMPROMISING RIGOUR
Faugier states that: 'The practice of nursing cannot be open to any compromise in the standards of care for individual patients and this should be reflected in the supervisory process' (1996: 62). With this in mind, she advocates that the supervisory style should be one of uncompromising rigour.

TRUST
Supervision is an intimate process. It would be foolish to ignore the possibility that this intense and professionally personal relationship can produce a sense of closeness and bonding between supervisor and supervisee. Although some writers would argue about the reality of the situation, it cannot be denied that it will seem extremely real to either both or one of the parties concerned at the time.

Faugier suggests that inexperienced supervisees can misinterpret interest and concern on the part of the supervisor as something much more personal, and respond with open feelings of love or sexual attraction. This will challenge the supervisor who must handle the situation in a way that leaves no room for doubt about the intention of retaining strictly professional boundaries without embarrassing or hurting her supervisee.

What do supervisees want from supervisors?
The working relationship between the clinical nurse supervisor and her supervisee may be considered to be the most significant aspect of the entire process. I see it as the metaphorical 'oil' that greases the 'cogs' of the activity itself and which allows it to move forward smoothly and without friction or having the whole process seize up. Health professionals helping patients with psychological problems have long surmised that the very nature of the professional relationship itself can be as helpful to the patient as any particular model of therapy that might be used.

A problem for nursing supervision is that information on the essential ingredients of a 'good' supervisory relationship – especially from the position of the supervisee – is currently limited. Sloan (1996) states that although policy statements on clinical supervision advocate that supervisees should be encouraged to choose their own supervisor, little has yet been done to clarify exactly which supervisor characteristics are valued by potential supervisees. Sloan argues that although the professional relationship between the supervisor and her supervisee may be regarded as 'the key to effective clinical supervision', nursing research has yet to identify and evaluate the key elements that make the relationship work well. Sloan identified some nursing research that clarified what it is that supervisees want from their clinical supervisors. Although inconclusive, it may offer supervisors food for thought about what they can do to enhance the working relationship between themselves and their supervisees.

A survey of sixty-one clinical supervisors working in mental health nursing identified a range of activities carried out by those supervisors that were considered to be important to, and valued by, their supervisees. The specific activities included:

- Giving specific ideas about intervention
- Providing feedback on performance
- Creating a warm and supportive relationship
- Promoting autonomy
- Being competent (as a nurse)

(Pesut and Williams, in: Sloan, 1996)

Sloan states that specific activities of someone considered to be a 'good' supervisor, by their own supervisees, have been identified by several researchers and include:

- Allowing supervisees to observe their supervisor's clinical practice
- Utilising role-play during supervision to demonstrate interventions
- Providing relevant literature
- Encouraging the use of acquired skills
- Offering guidance with treatment and direction with interventions
- Providing a supportive relationship

(Sloan, 1996: 44)

What needs to happen before clinical supervision can begin?

Before clinical supervision can begin, either on an organisational or individual basis, a range of functions and criteria will need to be taken into consideration. Without due consideration in advance to the questions of how, where, when and why supervision will take place, the process is left open to a large number of potential pitfalls.

VIEWING CLINICAL SUPERVISION FROM TWO VIEWPOINTS
I find it helpful to think about these considerations in two main ways, namely:

- The extended viewpoint on clinical supervision
- The restricted viewpoint on clinical supervision

I will consider these in the next section.

The extended viewpoint on clinical supervision – looking at the big picture

The extended viewpoint on clinical supervision is used to examine clinical supervision from the perspective of the nursing organisation as a whole. It can be used to consider the feasibility and viability of clinical supervision in terms of all the nurses within that organisation and also offer the opportunity to consider ways in which it might be implemented, generally, throughout the organisation. Some of the questions that may be raised from taking this view and which potential supervisors and supervisees may want to ask of their nursing organisation can include the following below.

Does the organisation have a policy regarding clinical supervision of nurses?
If so, where is it? Who devised it? Does it need to be updated and/or revised? Who should you talk to about it? Can you – and others – offer to draw up such a document if it does not already exist?

If my organisation does not have a written policy, does it have a 'position' on clinical supervision?
What is the organisational position – is it generally positive or generally antagonistic towards the implementation of a clinical

supervision strategy? If antagonistic, what are the main reasons against implementing supervision at present. Is it an 'official' position (i.e. has it been formally ratified and documented) or is it of a more 'unofficial' nature (i.e. perhaps a widely known view of one or two senior executives) and therefore possibly more amenable to concerted pressure.

Does my organisation wish to implement clinical supervision for nurses?

If so consider what needs to happen before clinical supervision can be implemented? A useful starting point could be the formation of a steering-group or working party with terms of reference that might include the following considerations:

DEVISING A STRATEGY FOR IMPLEMENTATION OF CLINICAL SUPERVISION
Who is it for?
How often should it be offered?

FINDING AN APPROPRIATE NUMBER OF SUITABLY SKILLED AND TRAINED CLINICAL SUPERVISORS
Who should be invited to act as clinical supervisors?   A decision needs to be made around whether only nurses above a certain grading and/or experience will be invited to act as supervisors. It would also be useful to consider the demographical considerations of the organisation to ensure that, especially when the organisation covers a large area – perhaps even several towns – the selection does not become 'top-heavy' in any one sector.

Who will allocate supervisors to supervisees?   A department within the nursing organisation, and even a particular person within the department may be nominated to be responsible for the allocation of supervisees to supervisors. Large and diverse nursing organisations may wish to consider placing the responsibility for clinical supervision allocation within the post-registration training department (or equivalent), given supervision's links with skills development in the minds of many nurses. Organisations offering specific mental health nursing services may feel that their community or psychotherapy departments are also closely – and traditionally – associated with the practice of supervision, and there may well be a larger number of nurses experienced in receiving and offering clinical supervision in those departments.

How will supervisees be matched to supervisors?   A useful device to assist the allocation of clinical nurse supervisors, operated by an increasing number of nursing organisations, is a clinical supervision 'directory' or 'register'. Basically, this is a regularly updated document containing essential information on the clinical nurse supervisors trained and/or approved by the organisation, and perhaps widely circulated throughout the organisation, or kept within a particular department, according to local preference. Once compiled, the document can be made available to all nurses seeking supervision, who can then contact the supervisor directly, or via the clinical supervision co-ordinator, again depending on the organisational preference. There are various methods of compiling such information and each nursing organisation will have its own particular requirements that will ultimately determine the design of the 'register'. If the register is kept in loose-leaf, or plastic sheet form, individual forms can be added, removed and updated easily and simply. I offer my own example of a page from a clinical supervision register, below, which includes many of the key elements of such a document.

DECIDING WHAT TRAINING WILL BE REQUIRED FOR CLINICAL SUPERVISORS

Will training be offered 'in-house', by the organisation itself, or is there access to existing formal clinical supervision training from a local education provider? Many nurse education providers are now beginning to offer training modules and/or workshops in clinical supervision skills. How much training needs to be offered and what are the *essential* components should be another important consideration. Although there is a danger that prospective supervisors can be offered too little training, and consequently be sent off unprepared for the task, it can also be argued that there is a point past which training becomes superfluous to requirements when supervisors become too embroiled in the process of training for supervision to have the time or energy left to practise.

Those responsible for the strategic planning of supervision within organisations need to decide what will be the essential elements required by supervisors. A useful bench-mark could be to ensure that, as a minimum, all supervisors are trained in

Clinical Supervision Register Supervisor Information Sheet			
Name of Supervisor:	*Roberta Stevens*		
Areas of Nursing Practice:	*Community, Palliative Care*	Can supervise at supervisee's base?	*possibly*
Qualifications:	*RGN, ENB 237, ENB 998, Dip.N. (District Nursing), BSc (Hons)*		
Clinical Grade:	*Grade G*	Can offer group facilitation?	*no*
Other Professional Interests:	*Complementary Therapy*		
Supervision Training:	*'Introduction to Supervision' 15 credit module, Kleever College, May 1999.*	Method of Initial contact?	*Via clinical supervision organiser: ext. 2134*
Number of Previous Supervisees:	*2 (since January 1998)*		
Preferred Supervision Method/Style:	*'6 – Eyes' model*		

Figure 3.1 *Example of clinical supervision register sheet*

basic communication and listening skills, have an understanding of reflective practice and an awareness of appropriate models of clinical supervision. Training is essentially pointless without assessment, however, and personnel responsible for organising and monitoring the training of supervisors within the organisation, should have a method of determining when the candidates have met – or have failed to meet – criteria designed to assess their level of understanding of training material. This advice may be more pertinent when the supervision training is 'in-house' and self-styled by the organisation, than when it is offered by an accredited education-provider.

Developing a system of clinical supervision in a nursing organisation

Bond and Holland (1998) offer a six-stage model for the development of a system of clinical supervision within nursing organisations, which they have based on original principles of supervision development offered by Kohner (1994), Swain (1995) and the UKCC (1996).

The strategy proposed by Bond and Holland (1998: 216–28) consists of six main stages. Because this strategy takes a more multi-disciplinary approach to clinical supervision than is offered here, I have occasionally adjusted the emphasis to the singular practice of nursing.

1   Information-sharing
    The tasks involved in this first stage of the strategy include:
    a)   Investigating the level of interest and expertise in clinical supervision currently existing within the organisation.
    b)   Convening a working group of interested personnel and including as many experienced clinical nurse supervisors as possible.
    c)   Encouraging working group members to share written material that is considered especially pragmatic and workable.
2   Skills training
    Consideration of what training is required, for whom and the most cost-effective form of obtaining it.
3   Decision about mode and structure
    Consideration of the form(s) of clinical supervision (including individual, 'facilitated group' or 'peer group' supervision) that will be offered within the nursing organisation.
4   Pilot
    Testing of the modes and overall strategy of clinical supervision through the use of a pilot scheme. Offer short periods of clinical supervision (three to six sessions) to a selected number of nurses within the organisation. Bond and Holland (1998) state that criteria for success of the clinical supervision strategy can be developed by researching the views of the pilot participants with questions such as: 'What exactly would be happening to tell you that it (clinical supervision) was a success?'
5   Evaluate, redesign
    Evaluate the success potential of the planned strategy for clinical supervision through examination of the responses from those nurses participating in the pilot scheme. Consider a redesign of the whole strategy or part of the strategy, according to the results of the pilot scheme.

6 Establish and monitor
   Establish the strategy following the clarification and implementation of any redesign deemed necessary after considering
   the finding of the pilot scheme. Some of the methods used for
   the evaluation stage of the strategy can be adapted as tools to
   monitor the progress and development of the full scheme.
   Bond and Holland suggest that 'the all-important sponsorship
   by a senior manager of the on-going clinical supervision
   system need to continue to be high profile and explicit in its
   support for the staff, as they continue to refine and develop
   their clinical supervision' (Bond and Holland, 1998: 227–8).

The restricted viewpoint on clinical supervision – attending to the nitty-gritty

The restricted viewpoint on clinical supervision assumes that the
organisation is in general agreement with the notion of clinical
supervision and has implemented a basic strategy for its delivery.
The phrase is used, therefore, to consider the operation of clinical
supervision from the viewpoint of the actual practitioner, who
will be more concerned with the minutiae of the practice than the
political and organisational considerations that will be 'seen'
when observing supervision from the extended viewpoint.

Once an overall agreement and strategy on the implementation
of clinical supervision within the nursing organisation has been
reached, a considerable number of small, but vitally important,
decisions will also need to be made to ensure a smooth transition
from its conception to its inception.

Solving the practical problems of clinical supervision

There is often a direct correlation between the amount of time
spent dealing with seemingly minor considerations and the
resulting enormity of the sense of achievement and success with
clinical supervision. If not enough time is spent on addressing
seemingly minor details – such as not booking the use of the
intended supervision room, and finding it in use as you arrive
with your first supervisee – it can ruin weeks of planning.

Below, I have raised some practical questions that can arise for
supervisors when they are looking at clinical supervision from the
restricted viewpoint, together with my own answers. They are

given with the cautionary note that, what works in one nursing organisation may well fall flat in another. At the very least, they may offer a starting point from which solutions may evolve – and ultimately, any solution or idea that is tailored-made to fit a specific problem has a greater chance of success than one taken straight 'off-the-peg'.

THE QUESTIONS OF TIME

- For how long should each supervision session last?
- How frequently should supervision occur?

The questions of how long each session lasts and how frequently they occur are crucial considerations that need to be decided and then carefully adhered to from the very first session. The answers will often depend on a number of factors including organisational constraints; the amount of clinical work each supervisee is bringing to the sessions and whether the supervisee will be seen alone or in a group. It is also too early in the development of nursing supervision to examine the choices practitioners are making about time spent in supervision, for definitive solutions to the problems.

Some nursing organisations, however, are opting for clinical supervision meetings that last for one hour per session and occur once every four weeks. This is a useful starting point for consideration, at least in terms of how realistic it may be for you as a participant and the organisation, generally.

Perhaps the most useful advice is that the length and frequency of supervision sessions should be based, as far as possible on:

- An objective overview of the needs of the supervisee
- The availability of the supervisor
- The constraints and existing policies of the organisation

THE QUESTIONS OF PLACE

Where will the clinical supervision take place?   This important question warrants careful consideration from two main perspectives. Firstly, from the more obvious logistical angle of whether or not there will be enough available space in the supervisor's office or ward to conduct regular clinical supervision there. Is where you regularly work too busy or too noisy to consider making it the venue for supervision? Secondly, consider the question from the point of view of the supervisee. Does he feel able to visit *your* place of work on a regular basis? This needs to be considered on several levels, but I would suggest, chiefly to look at it logistically. Will he need to make a long journey that could become impracticable or does he know some of your colleagues, or worse, does he work with them? This might lead to difficulties in the supervisee feeling safe enough to speak openly during the supervision session.

Do you have a room of your own to use or will you need to find one? In some nursing organisations, the supervisor will travel to the supervisee, which could, again, lead to difficulties in creating a confidential and 'safe' place. If the supervisor has a room of her own strategically situated away from clinical areas, this could solve that problem.

Can you have the same room at the same time on a regular basis or will you need to book different ones? Having to book rooms for each separate session can lead to confusion and disruption of the sessions if it is not properly managed. The supervisee needs to feel that he is being attended to by the supervisor and that his needs are paramount, at least for the time set aside for *his* clinical supervision.

If it is necessary to book different rooms for each supervision session, try to do it for the whole year, or another considerable 'block' of time, and not from one session to another. Giving this block of dates to your supervisee, in order that he knows where he will be several weeks in advance can go a long way to establishing a sense of containment and assurance in the supervisee.

Can you eliminate or reduce the prospect of interruption? It is import- ant that you do everything possible to ensure that you will not be inappropriately disturbed during the supervision session. Interruptions can come from so many different places – often all at once – that it will be difficult to prepare for all of them, but it is important that, as a clinical supervisor you consider that for the period of the supervision session it is your number one priority other, perhaps, than for certain very specific and predetermined events for which you are prepared to be contacted. If there are issues that you consider important enough to be contacted about during supervision sessions, make sure you have a clear idea about what these are and tell whoever is likely to contact you, well in advance.

Think about . . . reasons to be interrupted during clinical supervision

1 Write a list of all the issues, concerns and situations that you would wish to be contacted about *during* a clinical supervision session even though this would interrupt the session.
2 Take out of this list all of those things that could result in serious consequences for yourself or others if you were not made aware of them within one hour of their occurrence.
3 Consider this second list: Does it contain everything that you want to be interrupted for? If so, think about giving it to whoever should let you know if one of the issues occur when you are supervising.

I would suggest that there is only one appropriate way to arrange to be contacted during a clinical supervision session. Designate someone to knock on the door when – and only when – one of the pre-stated situations arises. The conditions for the knock on the door may change and the person charged with the task also, from time to time, but if this arrangement can be made it will make supervisory life so much simpler for all concerned and allow the supervisor to disengage from some of the more intrusive forms of communication.

There are innumerable ways in which supervisors and supervisees can be disturbed during a clinical supervision session, and 'Power's Law of Uninvited Intrusion' holds that: If a clinical supervision session can be disturbed or disrupted – it will be! There are also several ways to avoid this happening, and the first is very 'low-tech' but extremely effective:

1 Hang a 'do not disturb' sign on the door
   A sign printed on A4 paper saying something to the effect of *'Clinical Supervision In Progress: Please Do Not Disturb'* should prevent disturbance from outside the room – but be warned that some pranksters have been known to knock on doors with such signs and ask politely if the occupant was aware that her Do Not Disturb notice was displayed! There is probably more potential, though, for disturbance from *within* the room itself and a number of possible sources will be to blame. My final two suggestions on how to avoid 'Power's Law of Uninvited Intrusion' are based on taking preventative action with not human, but mechanical and electronic, culprits in mind.

2   Unplug or divert the telephone
    If the room you are using does not have a telephone connected,
    so much the better. If it is not your room, and it does have
    a phone, consider disconnecting it for the duration of the
    supervision. When using your own room for a clinical super-
    vision session, arrange to divert calls received by your own
    telephone to a colleague or possibly an answering machine.
    Switch off the ringer, if possible. In order to remain credible in
    the eyes of your supervisees as a safe and containing super-
    visor, *never* answer the telephone during a supervision session
    even if the temptation to do so can often be very strong.
3   Switch off the beeping computer
    Modern technology has brought the nurse a range of com-
    munication devices other than the telephone including
    bleepers, pagers, fax machines, mobile telephones, radios
    and computers, that can be a boon in the right circumstances,
    but a considerable nuisance when the focus of attention
    should be a supervisee with limited time and a great deal to
    say. During a clinical supervision session, turn off the audible
    signal on pagers and mobile phones. Even setting them to
    vibrate rather than bleep, buzz or ring can be distracting and I
    would advise against it, if a voice mail facility is available on
    the device.

   I know of at least one clinical supervisor who leaves the e-mail
facility of her computer switched on when supervising. For much
of the time, this is of no real distraction and the computer sits
quietly on the desk with the 'screen saver' running. The screen
saver itself is of minimal distraction, but I would suggest that a
blank screen is infinitely less distracting. The real problem arises
when the computer 'beeps' to announce the arrival of new
electronic mail and the previously-focused supervisor is unable to
resist the temptation to nudge the 'mouse' to reveal the screen and
see what message just came in. This can be an extremely dis-
heartening message to the supervisee who is likely to conclude
that almost anything is more important to the supervisor than
what he may have to say.

Is the room comfortable?   The comfort of supervisor and supervisee
is important to ensure that they can concentrate on the task in
hand without having to be distracted by noise, heat, cold or some
other infuriating element.

Too much comfort, however, can be equally distracting from the task in hand. Avoid equipping the clinical supervision room with easy chairs, coffee machines and ash trays. Both parties need to concentrate and focus on the supervisory task in no less a way than they would on direct work with patients.

The supervisor and supervisee are not coming together for the kind of relaxed chat that might be expected in the staff room. Consequently, the accoutrements of post-work winding down – drinking, smoking and crashing-out in easy chairs – are not only inappropriate, but can seriously interfere with the serious business of supervision.

Will the room need to be re-arranged before supervision starts?   Why should the furniture in the clinical supervision room – and its arrangement – have any bearing on the progress or quality of the supervision itself?

Clinical supervision happens within the context of a conversation. In order to help that conversation flow the speakers need to feel that they are both free and able to speak, as openly as possible. If we accept that clinical supervision is not a managerial exercise with the supervisee in a one-down position from the supervisor, it follows that whatever can be done to reflect the equality of the participants is vital to a successful outcome.

There are a variety of ways in which the supervisor can set out the chairs in which she and the supervisee will sit for the clinical supervision session. The choice of seating arrangement that she makes can have a considerable bearing on how the professional relationship develops in the future, and so the choice of seating plan that she employs needs to be given careful consideration.

If there is a desk in the room – and most offices in nursing organisations will be furnished with at least one or two, probably occupying around half of the overall room space – its potential for effecting the supervisory relationship can be great and the supervisor should not make the initial mistake of underestimating its influence. Desks, and how the seating is arranged around them, can say a great deal about both the person who uses it the most often, and his/her relationship to and view of the people that he/she meets around it.

A story of intrusive furniture – the entrepreneur and his big desk   While studying at college in the early 1970s, I was employed as a garage attendant during the evenings and weekends. The garage was owned by a local entrepreneur who was not afraid to express his pride at being a self-made millionaire – he wore designer clothes, and drove expensive sports cars adorned by glamorous women, and was treated with a great deal of respect, if not to say awe, by many of his employees and local people, some of whom spoke of him in hushed tones and regaled him with a celebrity-like status.

My view, on first seeing him, was that this person was not necessarily perturbed by the local perception of himself. My insight that he may have actually *encouraged* it was only gained, however, on the morning that I was invited to meet him at his headquarters in the town. I was ushered into an office that had, in the centre, quite the largest oak desk that I have seen outside the boardrooms of the wealthier hospital Trusts. Not only was this desk extremely large and imposing, it was raised up about twenty-four inches from the floor on a wooden plinth. There was no chair on the visitor's side of this desk, nor was there any way around it to sit next to its occupant who – with the effect of having to crane my neck slightly to look at him far across the other side of this vast sea of dark oak – became so imposing that it was difficult to remember why I had been summoned in the first place. There is no doubt in my mind that this man knew exactly what effect his desk had on those that entered the inner sanctum of his office. No one was ever in any doubt just who was the boss!

Four seating arrangements and a desk   Anyone who wants to feel important and superior should find the biggest desk possible and sit themselves squarely behind it. Preferably leaving the hapless interviewees to stand at the other side looking upwards in awe and wonder. Any clinical nurse supervisor who wishes to establish a meaningful and fruitful professional relationship with her supervisee in a room that contains a large desk should consider alternative strategies for its inclusion in the supervision process.

A seating strategy that I call the 'conversational arrangement' requires two chairs to be placed at one corner of the desk, at right angles to each other. This has the effect of giving both supervisor and supervisee an area of the desk on which to lean, or place their notes and with the added advantage of a largely unobstructed view of each other. The distance placed naturally between the two people when seated in this arrangement, is often a comfortable one – being neither too close to each other nor too far away – but this also can be easily adjusted by one or both moving along the desk. I would strongly recommend this seating arrangement whenever the supervision room is occupied by a large desk.

If at all possible, the supervisor should avoid arranging the seats directly across the desk from each other. I refer to this as the 'bank-manager arrangement' and it will, no doubt, be familiar to everyone who has ever met a bank manager to discuss an overdraft or found themselves in a similarly business-like situation. It is also very familiar to nurses who have met senior colleagues in formal and often stressful or difficult circumstances – such as applying for a new post, being appraised or even reprimanded. In any such situation, it is possible that the person on the 'wrong' side of the desk felt intimidated, insecure or even threatened. The presence of the imposing desk between him and his interviewer is unlikely to have helped to alleviate these feelings – and it may have even enhanced them. The clinical nurse supervisor should do what she can to ensure that any sense of intimidation and threat in the supervisee is reduced to a minimum and that he is not left feeling that he is taking part in a formal interview.

The 'coffee-table arrangement' is a seating plan that I would recommend whenever it is possible for the supervisor and her supervisee to sit away from a large desk, and when there is another small table – such as an occasional table or a coffee-table – available in the room. A small table placed between two chairs can give the sense of a 'boundary' between the two people without the sense of an imposing barrier that is often experienced from sitting across a large desk. It may be possible to place a plant or small ornament on this table or – more practically – it can be used to conveniently place a small clock or a watch between the supervisor and her supervisee, should there not be one on the wall, which they can both use to gauge the amount of time still available to them in the session.

Two chairs placed near each other without a small table between them can also be a satisfactory seating arrangement, and one that is still preferable, in my view, to the bank-manager arrangement. It is possible though, that those supervisors who recant to the 'no-table arrangement' having used the 'coffee-table' arrangement, may find themselves almost inexplicably wondering why they feel somewhat disconcerted by what now appears to be a gaping chasm between themselves and their supervisee.

Think about . . . some ways to arrange seating around a desk or table

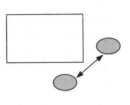

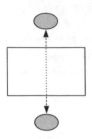

1 The conversational arrangement   2 The bank-manager arrangement

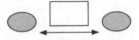

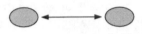

3 The coffee-table arrangement   4 The no-table arrangement

In the four diagrams above, the spheres represent the clinical nurse supervisor and her supervisee as seated on chairs. In the first two diagrams, the large rectangles represent a desk in the room being used for clinical supervision. In the third diagram the small rectangle represents a small 'occasional' or coffee-table placed between the two chairs. There is no table at all between the chairs in the fourth diagram.

1   What will be the particular influence that each of the four seating arrangements has on the process of the clinical supervision?
2   Is any one seating arrangement likely to have a more positive or negative impact on the clinical supervision session than another?
3   Is there a seating arrangement here that you do – or would – prefer to use when talking to colleagues? What are the advantages of that arrangement for you and for your colleagues? What are the disadvantages of that arrangement?
4   Is there a seating arrangement above – or similar – that has been utilised when a clinical supervisor or another colleague has been talking with you? Think about the topic of that conversation. Was the seating arrangement appropriate to the discussion? Did it influence how you felt about your colleague and the discussion itself?

Should clinical supervision be mandatory for nurses?

The UKCC *Position Statement on Clinical Supervision* (1996) endorses: '. . . the establishment of clinical supervision in the interests of maintaining and improving standards of care, in an often uncertain and rapidly changing health and social care environment.' The position statement also makes clear the UKCC view that 'every practitioner should have access to clinical supervision'.

There is a clear intention here, that clinical supervision for nurses becomes widely implemented across the nursing spectrum as regularly as possible, by the majority of practising nurses. But does that equate to a recommendation that the practice becomes one that nurses are *required* to undertake as part of their professional activities? And, if not, why not?

The official position
When this book went to print, the UKCC had not advocated that clinical supervision become a mandatory activity for nurses. The official view – embodied in the UKCC Position Statement on clinical supervision – is that: 'Clinical supervision is not to be a statutory requirement for nurses and health visitors. This position may be reviewed if the need arises' (UKCC, 1996).

I would suggest that although there is scope for change to this position, it is unlikely to occur in the near future. There are those who advocate the use of a more proactive stance on the part of the UKCC and feel that clinical supervision for nurses will be left to 'the fate of the winds' (Farrington 1996), without a more imposing approach to the implementation of supervision in nursing.

The case for mandatory supervision
The pro-mandatory supervision lobby argue that nurses will never become the true professionals that they aspire to be unless they receive supervision, with all its benefits of support and education, as a professional *right* and not a punitive measure aimed at bringing the wayward into line. They further argue that the introduction of supervision in nursing is currently too sporadic and piecemeal to have any real effect. Farrington (1996) offers one such succinct argument in favour of mandatory clinical supervision for nurses:

> Talking about 'light touch management influence' is not particularly helpful to a stressed workforce which is intent on being valued, treated equitably, paid its worth and being supported clinically. The rhetoric of management is not what is required, and leaving supervision to the fate of the winds is not the way forward. As we move into the next century nursing in Britain needs clear messages of leadership and direction. (Farrington, 1996: 716)

Dimond (1998) argues that any nursing organisation could decide to include clinical supervision in the contracts of new staff, or amend existing contracts as part of local contract renegotiations. In this case, it could be agreed that a nurse might receive supervision on a regular basis or a more senior nurse might agree to include acting as supervisor for a maximum number of staff as part of their contractually defined nursing role.

The case against mandatory supervision

I would argue against the notion of mandatory clinical supervision in nursing on the grounds that it would ultimately lead to discontent and, in some instances, a state of going-through-the-motions. I add to this, my contention that human beings – and nurses are no exception – will instinctively, initially resist anything that is foisted upon them. It would, perhaps, be wiser to allow nurses to choose to be supervised while at the same time pro-actively encouraging its provision as widely as possible in all areas – both professional and geographic. While I fervently agree with Farrington that all nurses should have the *right* to be supervised, I would suggest that so long as nurses retain the right *not* to receive clinical supervision, they are better placed to – ultimately – choose what I see as the more positive option.

What are the legal implications of clinical supervision?

Potentially, there are a number of legal considerations to be made when setting up clinical supervision within a nursing organisation. These considerations are discussed with the proviso that they are issues which should be applied directly to a specific organisational or individual situation, rather than being taken as universally applicable pronouncements.

I will consider, here, the legal position in an important area of clinical supervision for nurses – professional accountability – and a second area – access to records – will be discussed in Chapter 5.

Professional accountability

In terms of professional accountability there are four main areas which have been outlined by Dimond that are relevant from the position of the supervisor particularly, but which may also have a bearing for her supervisee. These areas are:

- Reporting dangers
- Giving negligent advice
- Principles of law
- Duty of care to patients under the clinical care of the supervisee

REPORTING DANGERS

Clinical supervisors, according to Dimond, have a professional and contractual duty to make their concerns known about any supervisee who may be disclosing behaviour that may be considered dangerous or potentially dangerous to patients. In the United Kingdom, the UKCC may wish to consider professional conduct proceedings against nurses registered with them who fail to pass on relevant information regarding dangerous and unprofessional conduct to the appropriate persons within the nursing organisation in the first instance.

GIVING NEGLIGENT ADVICE

Although advice-giving is not, and should not, ever be considered the primary aim of clinical supervision for nurses, it would be foolish to ignore the possibility that some clinical nurse supervisors, at some point in their careers, may fall into the trap of offering their supervisees advice. Dimond (1998) points out that:

> . . . if inappropriate or negligent advice were given to the supervisee there would be a possibility that the supervisor could be held liable. Also, if harm befell the supervisee as a result of following this advice, he/she might seek compensation from the employer for the negligence of employees acting in course of employment (vicarious liability). (1998: 487)

PRINCIPLES OF LAW

In connection with the notion of negligent advice, Dimond points out that: '. . . it is a principle of law that liability can exist if a person is reliant upon advice which, if given negligently, causes them harm'. In explaining this principle of law, Dimond refers to the legal case of Headley Byrne and Co Ltd vs Heller and Partners Ltd (1964) and states that there are four elements which must be present before this principle can be established. These elements are:

1 A duty of care which arises from a special relationship between the parties such that one realises that the other is likely to rely upon any advice which is given

2   Advice which is given negligently or without due care
3   Reliance upon that advice
4   Harm arising from the reliance

Dimond states that all of these elements could arise in the relationship between a clinical nurse supervisor and her supervisee. If the supervisor could prove exemption from liability, this might be accepted in the situation where the supervisee, acting on the advice of the supervisor, might have caused loss or damage to property. Such an exemption would not be valid however, if the supervisee's actions, as a consequence of his supervisor's advice had been responsible for personal injury or death – under the Unfair Contract Terms Act 1977. Dimond suggests that any employer of a clinical nurse supervisor could be held vicariously (indirectly) liable for prosecution themselves, even if they contractually prohibit that supervisor from giving advice, as that advice is likely to be regarded by the courts as being given in the course of employment in spite of the prohibition.

DUTY OF CARE TO PATIENTS
Dimond states that:

> A situation could arise were the clinical supervisor becomes aware that the supervisee is dangerous to a patient . . . and fails to take any action. When the patient is harmed by the practitioner it may become apparent that the clinical supervisor was in the position of being able to take action to prevent the harm arising. (1998: 487)

She argues that in this case the supervisor's employer could be held vicariously liable for the negligence in view of the fact that the supervisor owed a duty of care to the patient. Similarly if a practitioner witnesses an activity that is likely to cause harm, the failure to prevent that harm occurring could be regarded as professional misconduct.

4

Communicating in Clinical Supervision

Key issues in this chapter

- Communication and clinical supervision
- Non-verbal communication in supervision
- Verbal communication in clinical supervision
- How to offer supervision feedback
- How supervisees can respond to feedback

Communication and clinical supervision

Communication is the essence of clinical supervision. Supervisors and supervisees need to talk to each other in a way that is focused, meaningful and productive. Because clinical supervision for nurses is about more than a pleasant chat over a coffee, it requires a more formalised – and skilled – approach from the clinical supervisor.

It is important for clinical nurse supervisors to be aware of a range of intervention techniques that should result in a clinical supervision that has clarity, direction and purpose. The more awareness that the supervisor has of the many ways in which her supervisee may tell her something, the more likely she will be to get the message.

The key elements of communication

In order for any message to be sent and received, certain key elements are involved. In a simple model of communication these elements can be described as:

- Sender (encoding thought/emotion processes)
- Message (content and channel)

- Noise
- Receiver (decoding message)
- Feedback (encoding thought/emotion processes)

The communication process begins when the *sender* decides that he wishes to communicate his thoughts and/or feelings with the *receiver*. He then needs to decide not only on the *content* of *message* he wishes to send but also what *channel* that message will take. In some communication models, the process of choosing a channel for the message – whether this is the spoken word, the written word or a non-verbal gesture (perhaps sending a bunch of flowers or slapping someone in the face) – is referred to as *encoding*. When these choices are made (and assuming that the sender has not chosen to abandon the process), the message can be sent. The receiver then needs to *decode* the message before it can be fully understood. The processes involved in decoding a message may include listening to spoken words, reading a letter, feeling a physical contact, taking receipt of a gift or any other of a number of actions involving one or more of the receiver's senses. Once the message has been decoded the receiver can choose to send a message of her own. The process is identical to that begun by the sender – the receiver has thoughts and/or feelings about the sender, decides what message she wishes to send, chooses an appropriate channel, encodes the message and sends it. An important difference, here, is that the receiver's message now becomes *feedback*, which the sender can use to determine how the receiver has responded to his original message. This feedback will then help the receiver to decide if he should send another message and the content and channel he should use. The process of two-way communication has begun.

Think about . . . channels of communication

1   Write a list of some things that someone could do (either knowingly or unknowingly) in order that you become aware that they are:
    a) In love
    b) Excited
    c) Worried
    d) Irritated
2   What channels of communication can be best used to tell someone:
    a) You love them
    b) They are being made redundant
    c) You are annoyed with them
    d) They have made a serious clinical error

Interference in communication

An important later addition to some models of communication is the notion of *noise* – the recognition of interference to the message before it is encoded by the receiver. In its simplest form, the concept of noise might suggest that the sender is speaking in a language that the receiver cannot fully understand, or that the receiver mishears a certain word that totally changes the fundamental nature of the message. Interference from noise might be increased by the psychological conditions of the receiver at the time of the message. She may be drunk or under the influence of drugs, or she may have particularly strong feelings towards the sender of the message – either positive or negative – which may interfere with her reception of the message.

Think about . . . noisy communication

Read the following story and then identify the specific elements that might have interfered with and distorted the original message from the nurse to Frank. Try to include psychological, physical and social factors that might have influenced both the sender and receiver.

When, in his late fifties, Frank was admitted to hospital for heart surgery, he quickly struck up an acquaintance with Harold in the next bed, who was also awaiting surgery – but which to Frank had seemed of a much more serious nature, despite Harold's optimistic view of the outcome and his very high regard for the medical and nursing care he was receiving. The two men only had a day to discover that they had much in common – their experiences in the army, at work, their personal interests as well as their shared concerns about their current health problems – before Harold was moved to an adjoining ward. Frank heard no more of Harold for a few days and his thoughts quickly became caught up in the preparations for his surgery. The operation went well, and Frank had spent two days recovering, when he looked at the empty bed next to his and remembered Harold. 'What happened to Harold?', he asked an obviously too-busy nurse as she hurried past him one morning, carrying charts and case-notes. 'Who? Oh, Mr Jones . . . oh . . . he's gone' she offered in a way that seemed like an apology to Frank, as she rushed towards the nursing-station. Frank was devastated. Gone? But he was so sure everything would be all right! He was so full of life. It was fortunate for Frank that the busy sender of the message that Harold had 'gone', knew something about the concept of noise in communication, and that she was also skilled enough as a nurse to reflect on her interaction with Frank, once she had disposed of her task in hand. The nurse returned to Frank's bedside just as he was contemplating sending a message of sympathy – using the channel of a card – to Harold's 'widow'. 'I'm sorry, Mr Smith, if I gave you the wrong idea earlier.' Frank looked up, puzzled as she continued, 'When I said that Mr Jones had "gone", I merely meant that he has recovered from his operation and that he has gone . . . home.'

Four basic principles of communication

Watzlawick et al. (1967) described four basic principles of communication theory, which can inform the process and assist clinical nurse supervisors to understand and utilise the essential – and possibly unavoidable – elements of communication to the ultimate benefit of the supervision relation generally, and the supervisee specifically.

1   ONE CANNOT *NOT* COMMUNICATE

There is a message in everything that we do. There is, equally, a message in the things that we do not do. If someone greets me with a smile, I may reasonably infer that the smiler is sending me the message that she is being friendly towards me. If I meet the same person again, but she does not smile at me, I may conclude that she is not sending me another 'friendly' message and that she may in fact be sending me a message of a completely different kind.

My friend, Peter, once sent flowers to Sarah, with a note inviting her for lunch. On the note, he had written the number of his answering machine with a polite instruction that should she wish to decline his offer, Sarah could simply call him to say 'no, thank you'. Peter never received a call nor any other verbal or written communication from Sarah. However, he most definitely *did* get the message! In this case I would regard Peter's flowers and written invitation as *direct communication*, and the absence of any response from Sarah as *indirect communication*. While non-action in response to an initial communication may be considered as indirect communication, it would be have been foolish for Peter to see it as no communication at all.

Ellis (1995) expands on the basic principle that we cannot *not* communicate by adding that once a message has been sent, it cannot be retracted. He makes the point that that it is virtually useless for us to follow an utterance or other form of message with 'did not say that' or 'ignore what I just did'. Once a message has been sent, it is irreversible. The receiver of the message may choose to ignore it or hear it in a different way than was originally intended, but any message that has been sent – whether it is as a result of direct or indirect communication – cannot be unsent.

2   EVERY COMMUNICATION HAS A CONTENT AND RELATIONSHIP ASPECT SUCH THAT THE LATTER CLASSIFIES THE FORMER AND IS THEREFORE A META-COMMUNICATION

Who – and what – I am in relation to another person has an important bearing on how any message I send them is received and understood. If I say to my friend, who has just disclosed that she has made a small and inconsequential error of judgement: 'You are hopeless – what *will* I do with you?', she may well accept it as the playful and harmless comment that it was intended to be. If, on the other hand, I use exactly the same phrase with a junior colleague for whom I have managerial responsibility, he may regard it as a negative judgement of his professional ability and become justifiably concerned, if not aggrieved, as a result.

The relationship between the parties involved in sending and receiving a communication always has an effect on how that message is both sent and received. The underlying relationship becomes a communication in itself – sometimes called a meta-communication – that influences the reception of the spoken words, often irrespective of any tonal emphasis given to them. In this regard then, the maxim of: 'It's not what you say but how you say it . . .' changes to: 'It's not what you say but who you are when you say it that makes all the difference.'

Clinical nurse supervisors should consider it an important on-going task to concern themselves with how their relationship with the supervisee might be acting as a meta-communication that is influencing the messages that they are sending and receiving. Although the supervisor may wish for the most balanced and equitable professional relationship possible, it may be that her supervisee has a totally different perspective and it will ultimately be the supervisee's view of the supervision relationship that influences the meta-communication.

3   A SERIES OF COMMUNICATIONS CAN BE VIEWED AS AN
UNINTERRUPTED SERIES OF INTERCHANGES
No message exists in a vacuum. Most interchanges between indi-viduals, with the possible exception of initial greetings, have a *history* behind them and a *future* ahead of them.

Most supervisees meeting their clinical supervisor for the very first time will have gleaned some information, either by direct questioning of others that have met and/or worked with the super-visor, or through indirect methods such as hearsay and gossip. The supervisee will then be in the position of meeting his supervisor with some information – no matter how scant or inaccurate – stored about the supervisor which will influence how the supervisee hears what is said to him, from the very beginning of the relationship.

In extreme cases, one person may draw an entirely speculative conclusion about another which remains fixed no matter what that person says or does to contradict the assumption. The clinical nurse supervisor can find herself on the receiving end of a concept sometimes referred to as the 'halo effect', whereby anything she says or does is received in the light of the very favourable perception that the supervisee has allowed himself to have of her, from before they ever met.

4 ALL COMMUNICATION RELATIONSHIPS ARE EITHER SYMMETRICAL OR COMPLEMENTARY, DEPENDING ON WHETHER THEY ARE BASED ON EQUALITY OR INEQUALITY

A symmetrical communication relationship is one in which both parties to the communication are considered – by themselves and each other – to be of an equal status and position and neither party is considered to be more superior or inferior than the other.

A typical example of *symmetry* in communication would be in the case of two close friends; one of whom is still in training as a student nurse and is shortly to embark on a nursing career from close to the bottom of the professional ladder. The other is a head of nurse education, who has recently been awarded an MBE for services to nurse education. Despite this, these friends currently having widely different nursing roles at, arguably, opposite ends of the professional spectrum, they do not work together and their respective professional standings in no way affect their social interaction. Because they have been close friends for many years, and they do not meet in a work-setting, their communications are not affected by a power-differential that might be present if they were colleagues only and not friends. In essence, they regard themselves as equals and their communications are always symmetrical in nature.

However, when the head of nurse education meets with a nursing student training within her faculty, and with whom she does not have a personal friendship, the communication relationship is described as *complementary*, rather than symmetrical. The complementary relationship is affected by the power (and status) differential between the two people involved, and all of the communications between them will be affected by this factor in their relationship. It is very unlikely, for example, that within a complementary relationship the student nurse will be 'cheeky' or 'playful' with the head of nurse education as her friend the student nurse might be.

The clinical nurse supervisor needs to take regular stock of the actual and perceived relationship that is operating between herself and the supervisee. The supervision situation is complex in that, no matter how much the supervisor may wish for as symmetrical a relationship as possible with her supervisee, it will always have elements that render it as inevitably complementary in nature. The astute clinical nurse supervisor will be aware of when the relationship is being adversely affected by a swing too far in either direction.

How to send a message without saying a word

Newborn babies have not yet learned to speak or write. Yet their mothers frequently know when they are hungry or cold or uncomfortable or contented. The baby uses facial expression; the position of its body (including arm and leg movements) and sounds (gurgles, suckling sounds, crying and screaming) to often get across very definite messages of its state of unease or contentment. As the baby grows – although still not able to speak – it learns to use behaviour in order to communicate its needs in a more defined manner.

Although spoken and written forms of communication are becoming increasingly more advanced and complex, the clinical nurse supervisor needs to be aware of other ways in which people can communicate. If we are not aware of these more subtle methods, we may well miss some very important messages that are being sent our way.

The section below, adapted from the work of Argyle (1992) and Lieberman and Cobb (1987b), lists some of the body language that we may need to 'listen to' in clinical supervision together with a few suggestions to its possible meaning and a rough guide to ways in which supervisors can interpret and use this form of language. When you next listen to your colleagues, friends and supervisees try to listen with your ears (to the words), your eyes (to the behaviours and gestures) and your brain (to the context of the discussion and your relationship with the speaker), and decide if the words are now making more – or different – sense.

TYPES OF NON-VERBAL COMMUNICATION

Bodily Contact   This type of contact includes the whole gamut of possible human contact including: touching (hands, arms, knees), poking, hitting and rubbing parts of our bodies against another person.

Possible meanings Aggression; sexual interest, control (pushing, pulling, leading); symbolic gestures (patting on the back, stroking, shaking hands or holding hands) can convey intimacy.

Value to clinical supervision Physical contact with supervisees beyond – possibly – a handshake at the start of the first session is usually unnecessary and inadvisable. Physical contact from supervisee to supervisor should be noted together with the context within which it is displayed and discussed, if appropriate.

PHYSICAL PROXIMITY
How we stand and sit in relation to another person can be very telling of our relationship with them – whether currently experienced or desired.

Possible meanings This is often a clue – and also a cue – to intended intimacy. Its significance varies with the physical surroundings and the context of the relationship. People sitting or standing close together on a crowded train may have no such desire for intimacy with each other. Given a choice, however, people usually stand or sit closer to those they like and/or to whom they are sexually attracted. A change in proximity can be a clue to the wish to begin or end an encounter.

Value to clinical supervision Sit close enough to hear your supervisee comfortably. Try to angle the chairs to about forty-five degrees so that you are not sitting directly face-to-face.

ORIENTATION
The concept of orientation is connected to that of physical proximity but its use can result in the conveyance of more complex messages.

Possible meanings People will sit or stand differently in relation to the other person, depending what message is to be conveyed, or the circumstances of the meeting. A manager who sits in a chair that is higher or bigger than that offered to his staff may be signalling that he wishes to be treated as if superior to colleagues.

Value to clinical supervision If we imagine that in Figure 4.1, **X** is sitting at a table, we can see how **Y** can convey at least three different meanings depending upon where she sits in relation to

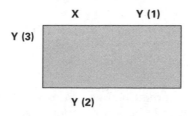

Figure 4.1   *Seating positions around a table*

X. In position (1), **Y** may be offering to co-operate with **X**, extend friendship or even develop intimacy (this is further determined by physical proximity and speech content during the meeting). Being seated in position (2), directly across the desk from **X**, **Y** may be preparing to formally interview **X**, reprimand him and/or express a conflicting viewpoint. In position (3), **Y** is best placed to hold a professional conversation or discussion with **X**, when both parties are seated near a table. The corner position offers a direct view and allows both people to comfortably write or refer to documents.

BODY POSTURE
How we stand, sit and walk can all help to convey certain messages, either knowingly or unwittingly, to others.

Possible meanings   Various messages can be conveyed. Distinctive postures include dominant (standing erect, hands on hips, head tilted back) and submissive (head bowed, shoulders slumped). Posture may also indicate: emotional state (wringing hands to indicate anxiety), attitude (turning your back on an adversary); styles of expression (folding arms across chest to indicate exclusion) and past or present roles in life (the erect bearing of an old soldier).

Value to clinical supervision   Supervisors should endeavour to maintain an open posture, in order not to discourage supervisees. Avoid folding arms across chest or turning body away from supervisee. Leaning slightly forwards toward supervisee and crossing legs towards them (which turns body in supervisee's direction) and sitting so that inside of wrists are upwards, can demonstrate a desire to engage with the supervisee.

GESTURES

Movements of the hands, feet and head can help to convey direct messages. They can also be involuntary movements of the body that are more ambiguous in meaning.

Possible meanings　Human beings can exhibit a variety of some-times seemingly meaningless body movements, especially when they are emotionally aroused. Feelings of anger, excitement, sad-ness, frustration and guilt – amongst others – can all cause an individual to display a range of hand, head, arm, foot and leg movements either singly or combined.

Value to clinical supervision　An angry or frustrated supervisee may speak quietly but give the game away with a clenched fist. Anxious supervisees may fidget in their seat, touch their face or play with hair or jewellery. Emotionally and/or physically tired supervisees may rub their eyes, wipe their forehead or yawn. Supervisors can use head nods to 'reinforce' what has been said to them, giving it credibility – a non-verbal 'yes' – thus encour-aging the supervisee to continue speaking. Similarly, supervisors can also use an occasional nod of the head to signal to a second supervisee to speak. Rapid head nodding might indicate that the supervisor herself – or another supervisee – wishes to say something.

EYE CONTACT

How we look at someone and for how long can be important clues to the contact we wish to make and the sort of messages that we intend to send to another person.

Possible meanings　Direct eye contact can indicate a range of feelings on the part of the subject (the person making contact) depending on the given circumstances and/or speech content. It is almost always experienced as a greater sense of intimacy between the participants. Staring into someone's eyes for a long period of time can mean one or more of several things: affection, aggression, curiosity – but usually indicates that the subject is holding feelings towards the object (the person being looked at). Glances can take the form of long or short looks at the object, and can be furtive or open, playful or more sinister in intent. They can be combined to form complex strategies of 'eye-play' that are best interpreted in the light of the prevailing circumstances and/or speech content.

Value to clinical supervision   Eye contact and eye movements can play an important part in sustaining the flow of supervision interaction. When the supervisee speaks he may move his head (up or around) to look directly at the supervisor, in order to obtain feedback or assurance that he is being 'attended' to. Supervisors can combine the last few words of a comment with a brief eye contact with the supervisee that will indicate that it is his turn to speak. This can be used especially effectively in group supervision.

APPEARANCE

When considering someone's appearance think about the clothes they wear – and how they wear them – make-up, hairstyle, jewellery, body ornaments – and also how people sit, stand, walk and talk.

Possible meanings   Generally, we human beings put a great deal of effort into controlling our personal appearance. How we look can act as a 'badge'; giving a message to the rest of the world about who we think we are and how we would like to be treated. We do this through the clothes that we wear (and when we wear certain clothes), hairstyles, make-up, body ornaments (rings, studs and other piercings) and plastic surgery are all used to project an image of ourselves to the world at large. Messages can be sent in very obvious and blatant ways – the punk with a spiked, purple mohican haircut and ear-studs may be giving off clear signals about his need for individuality. Other appearance messages can be more subtle. A woman wearing a coat buttoned to the top, on a hot summer's day at the beach might be expressing a difficulty with being 'exposed'.

Value to clinical supervision   The supervisee's appearance can be most significant when viewed in terms of how it may change over time. Signs of increased informality (taking off a tie, kicking off shoes before a meeting, for example) may indicate that the supervisee is feeling more comfortable in the supervisor's presence. If the supervisee's appearance becomes increasingly unkempt or his personal hygiene deteriorates, it may indicate that he is experiencing increased levels of stress.

ASPECTS OF SPEECH

It is often not so much what we say but how we say it that can make all the difference to the messages we send.

Possible meanings   We can change the meaning of a simple sentence with attention to aspects of vocal quality including: loudness, pitch (high/low voice), rate of speech (speed of the words, lack of pauses) and flow (hesitations, pauses, errm's). The pattern of conversational speech is always affected by non-verbal aspects which can be clues to the conversational relationship. Does one person speak more than the other and dominate the conversation? Is one person speaking more quickly or slowly than another? How soon after one person speaks does another start? Does one person interrupt another frequently? All of the above can guide us towards understanding the state of the relationship, but must be considered within the context of the conversation.

Value to clinical supervision   An anxious supervisee may talk faster and at a higher pitch than usual. An angry supervisee may talk more loudly than usual or – paradoxically – not want to talk at all. A sad or unhappy supervisee may talk more slowly and/or in a more subdued or hesitant manner than usual. Supervisors can use pauses to indicate a full stop and as a cue for the supervisee to speak. Putting stress on a particular word can provide emphasis and focus. Raising the pitch at the end of a sentence can indicate surprise/disbelief or that a statement is intended as a question and/or that it requires a response. Supervisees that demonstrate lots of speech errors (umms and ah's, stuttering, repetitions) may be stressed, unsure of their subject matter and/or using devices to create time to think.

The spoken language of clinical supervision

Through the use of statements in which she offers her personally 'owned' perception of the clinical situation being discussed – as opposed to firing a barrage of questions – the supervisor can take the supervision relationship from the level of an intimidating, unbalanced interview to what I will refer to as a *reflective conversation*. The reflective conversation should have an emphasis on personally focused statements which are offered in a less anxiety-ridden environment than is likely to be generated by a question-

and-answer session. It should, as a result, be more conducive to the generation and flow of supervision material.

An important aspect of any conversation is that the participants should feel safe enough to offer their views free from rejection and ridicule and, if necessary, to contradict or alter views put to them by other speakers. The more that a clinical supervisor can become adept at using personal statements, the more she will encourage the supervisee to offer his own perception of the situation, even though this might be at the risk of contradicting her.

The grammar of clinical supervision

Lieberman and Cobb (1987a) described a training in communication techniques – 'The Grammar of Psychotherapy' – that they developed in response to the task of teaching interviewing and interactional skills to medical trainees and junior doctors. They acknowledge that their methods are themselves derived from previous work by Maguire et al. (1978), Heron (1975) and Ivey and Simek-Downing (1980).

The teaching aims of the method devised by Lieberman and Cobb that I consider pertinent to clinical supervision for nurses include:

- Simple interview skills such as the collection of objective information, the communication of clear instructions and ways of structuring an interview.
- Complex psychological and interactional skills such as the ability to be sensitive to important psychological and emotional issues.
- The ability to circumvent or modify rigid attitudes.
- An awareness of the importance of the (nursing) relationship and the various factors that can modify this (Lieberman and Cobb, 1987a: 590 – my brackets).

The verbal micro-skills of clinical supervision

Lieberman and Cobb's communication skills training method is particularly influenced by the work of Ivey (1971) who 'trained students in the use of attending behaviour, minimal activity responses, verbal following behaviour, open enquiry, and reflection of feelings' (in Lieberman and Cobb, 1987b: 594).

Ivey used the term 'micro-skill' to describe the various and separate components of any verbal interaction. It is these micro-skills that I am interested in discussing, particularly in relation to their use by clinical nurse supervisors.

Table 4.1 *Adaptation of Lieberman and Cobb's 'microskills' (1987b), to clinical nurse supervision*

Asking questions	Non-verbal facilitation	Making statements
Non-leading Open	Sounds	Orientation/Introduction
Non-leading Closed	Silence	Encouraging/Empathic
Leading Open		Summarising
Leading Closed		Checking/Seeking Clarification
		Focusing/Scanning/Prompting
		Self-Revelation

Three main types of verbal interaction
The important verbal interactions used by a clinical nurse supervisor can be divided into three main groups. These are:

- Asking questions
- Non-verbal facilitation
- Making statements

Each of these three groups can then be further broken down to offer the supervisor a wide range of basic verbal interventions that she can usefully call upon to guide her into action with her supervisee. Table 4.1, above, outlines the three main groups of verbal interactions and their related verbal interventions and I will go on to discuss each main category and its sub-categories, in turn, giving examples of how the various interactions can be used in the clinical supervision situation.

Asking questions
No matter how strong the emphasis on reflective practice, there will always be a place for the judicious use of questions by the clinical nurse supervisor. In fact, I can see no way in which sufficient material can be gathered in order for the supervisor to have a full understanding of her supervisee's clinical work without the careful use of such interventions. Although questioning, per se, has got something of a bad press in certain clinical circles, I believe that questions can be a powerful and valuable tool in clinical supervision if used with forethought and discretion. The four categories of questions in the table above, and which I will detail below, all have their place in the verbal repertoire of a clinical nurse supervisor. Their effectiveness, however, will depend very much upon how skilful she is in determining the appropriateness of their use.

OPEN QUESTIONS
Open questions usually begin with words such as 'what', 'how', 'why' or 'could'. Two key points about open questions are that they can never be answered by a simple 'yes' or 'no', and their use should always be intended to encourage the supervisee to discuss the current topic in more depth. Open questions will often have the advantage of making the supervisee feel more at ease, as the discussion should begin to feel more like a two-way process than a question and answer session.

CLOSED QUESTIONS
Closed questions usually begin with words such as: 'is', 'are', 'do' and 'did'. Questioners using this form should not expect the answers they receive to be elaborated on, as they might with open questioning, and most closed questions will inevitably be responded to with a 'yes', 'no' or 'don't know' (or a similar remark indicating that the supervisee cannot – or will not – respond). Although closed questions are probably the most confining form available to a clinical supervisor, there is still potential for much productive use, providing that they are implemented carefully and with forethought.

NON-LEADING QUESTIONS
If a question is to be truly 'non-leading' it should not be phrased in any way that suggests that the questioner requires a certain answer. This is possibly the most difficult form of questioning to master and requires a good deal of preparedness in the clinical nurse supervisor to be surprised by what they may hear in response and as a result to perhaps undergo a review of their present thinking and strategies.

LEADING QUESTIONS
Leading questions are very popular with the legal profession. Anyone who has ever stood in the witness box, offering evidence during a court proceeding, may have faced the extremely difficult prospect of repelling a well-honed leading question. One specific purpose of a leading question is to suggest the answer that the questioner requires in the question itself – hence the use of the legal cliché 'I put it to you that . . .' at the beginning of many such interventions.

A trap that supervisors may find themselves in, through the inaccurate use of questioning is one that I call *asking while answering*. Its effect is often to cause the recipient to feel that he has no choice other than to agree with the questioner. 'You will stay for cup of tea and some cake, won't you?', is one commonly asked leading question that is unlikely to provoke much objection, but there are many other situations when the careless, or even deliberate, use of *asking while answering* can result in confusion and conflict. There is also much scope for the positive use of such questions, but they should not be asked without an opportunity for the supervisee to refute the questioner's implicit suggestions.

Using non-verbal facilitation
The phrase *non-verbal facilitation* applies to everything that the clinical nurse supervisor does in order to help her supervisee fully express himself – without the use of the spoken word. Too many clinical nurse supervisors starting out may worry that if they are not *talking* to the supervisee then their contribution is invalid. I would counter that concern with the argument there is much that can be done in supervision without using *words*.

Sometimes, in the clinical supervision relationship – and, indeed, in many other types of relationships – the use of words can be a hindrance to progress. The supervisor needs to find another way to facilitate the supervisee in his expression of his thoughts, in the most expedient way possible. If the supervisor feels that she needs to respond to everything that her supervisee says with a comment of her own, this can lead to a stilted and jerky exchange, often with one or both parties struggling to *say* something interesting or useful, in turn. The more that a clinical nurse supervisor can become confident in her use of non-verbal facilitation, the more expertise she will gain in demonstrating a wide range of communications without struggling to find the words.

The two main areas of non-verbal facilitation that I will discuss are: *sounds* and *silence*. Both of these forms of facilitation have their own special role to play in the development of a fluid and cogent clinical supervision relationship. However, they are also liable to be considered more unusual forms of supervision communication than the spoken word. Because of this, the new user may need to overcome personal concerns around feeling foolish in executing them, or worries that their use may not be as effective as actually *saying* something.

My advice would be for the supervisor starting out to do nothing that she considers to be totally out of character. Rather, she should spend some time thinking about what she is doing already with particular regard to the use of sounds and staying silent. What are the natural vocal sounds and pauses that she makes during everyday conversation? What does she intend to imply by them? Can she modify and control her use so that they have even more impact as non-verbal communications? If the supervisor starts by examining what comes naturally to her, and then links these actions to the clinical supervision setting, she will gradually begin to create an advanced repertoire of communication skills.

MAKING SOUNDS
I know of a clinical supervisor who claimed to be able to make a humming sound through pursed lips – best spelt as 'mmmm' – in such a way that it could imply over twenty different meanings to the supervisee. I am not sure if that particular supervisor's claim was strictly accurate, but the story does serve to underline the potential for expressing oneself without the use of words. With consideration, I suspect that few people would deny the capacity for a well-formed 'mmmm' to imply a range of responses including: surprise; delight; agreement; disagreement; disbelief and interest in what the speaker is saying.

Sounds such as 'mmmm', 'ummm' and 'hmmm' can be used to encourage the supervisee to continue with what he wishes to say, without the need for the supervisor to use words, which in themselves could be heard as an interruption or a cue for the supervisee to *stop* speaking. Other sounds such as 'ah-ha', 'hah-ah', and 'uh-huh', may also all have a place in helping the supervisor to convey a certain meaning without the need for a complex sentence.

Some writers on communication techniques would include very short words and phrases such as 'OK', 'yes' (or 'yep' or 'yeah'), 'I see', 'right' and 'go on' in the *sounds* category. I believe that there is a crossover with many people's vocal styles where such an utterance becomes amalgamated into more of an overall sound – with a generally acceptable meaning – than a phrase using clearly defined words. The problem with the use of such sounds by clinical nurse supervisors, as with any specific communication technique, is that they can be overused and become irritating or regarded as pointless by the supervisee. On the other hand, if sounds are used sparingly, with forethought and deliberate intent, they can have a viable place in helping to facilitate effective communication.

KEEPING SILENT

The careless or extended use of silence has the potential to be very damaging to the process of clinical supervision. Most supervisors would accept that sitting in silence for too long is, at best, a fruitless exercise and, at worst, harmful to the process. Long silences can be anxiety-provoking for the supervisee. Silences can also induce a sense of insecurity in him which is often coupled with the idea that his supervisor is 'stuck' for something to say. A very long silence might even suggest to the supervisee that his supervisor has chosen not to offer a contribution, which in itself can lead to a concern that the supervisor is disinterested in what the supervisee has to say and – ultimately – in supervising him.

The carefully controlled use of silence has much to offer the clinical nurse supervisor. If the supervisor can learn to pause before she speaks, she may contribute to the supervisee's capacity for reflection, by allowing him to dwell, albeit briefly, on the thoughts and feelings that have been generated by the words he has just spoken. If the supervisor 'jumps in' with words of her own as soon as the supervisee stops speaking – or if she encourages the supervisee to go on speaking – a valuable opportunity to reflect on the thoughts and feelings engendered could be lost forever.

Another useful application of silence, is that it allows the supervisor to avoid '*mis-directing the supervisee*'. I use this term to suggest that the supervisor has the potential to take her supervisee down a 'supervision road' that he is not yet ready to travel. When a supervisee finishes recounting a clinical situation, or responding to a comment about it, the supervisor may assume that he has no more to say on the matter. Too often, in my view, supervisees are taken off the topic that they wish to discuss, because the supervisor wrongly assumes that having paused for breath – or thought – the issue is finished with and a new one can be begun. A more subtle, but potentially serious error, that supervisors can make, is to use the gaps in the supervisee's discourse to ask a question or make a comment that may seem related to the issue in hand, but that in fact, misdirects the supervisee away from the point he wished to make or the thought that he had that would have enlightened his thinking around the specific issue.

If the supervisor aims to remain silent for between 4–10 seconds each time her supervisee finishes speaking, it can have the potential to allow the flow of new thoughts and new feelings on the matter in hand. Many supervisees will also be tempted to fill the silent void with words, in order to make themselves feel less uncomfortable. To help avoid this, the supervisor can practise using phrases like: 'lets just sit quietly and think about that', so that her supervisee can discover the advantages of silent reflection. Just how much silence is appropriate for any given situation is best determined through experience. This learning will be accelerated or arrested depending upon the supervisor's level of awareness of the supervisee's sensitivity to the material being discussed.

Remaining silent in supervision may be a particularly difficult technique to accomplish for supervisors who are convinced that 'not speaking is not-doing'. Without awareness of the need for silence supervisors run the risk of *'treading on the supervision silence'* which, as I describe below, can have a detrimental effect on the supervision process and the supervisee's learning experience.

Treading on the supervision silence   Many comedians have testified to the validity of the old show business maxim that 'the essence of good comedy is timing'. One useful aspect of timing – in both comedic and everyday exchanges – is that it allows for the development of the *pregnant pause*, a space between the words that can be filled with a sort of 'hopeful expectation' by the listener. When the words are finally delivered by the speaker, their impact is then even stronger than it might have otherwise been.

I remember one famous entertainer recounting a painful incident from his early career, which taught him a valuable lesson. In the early part of his career he worked in live theatre as a 'straight-man' – 'feeding' lines to a major musical-hall comedy star of the time. The entertainer, although always well-intentioned, was at that time still something of a novice in the world of show business, and had yet to become fully conversant with some of the essential elements involved in comedic delivery.

One evening, during a live stage performance, he offered his well-rehearsed 'feed-line' as usual and this was responded to by the star's comedy 'punch-line' – no doubt delivered with all of the flair and expertise that only a seasoned professional can muster. The audience roared with laughter and the star began to savour the moment. Unfortunately, in his eagerness to play his part well, the novice entertainer delivered his next 'feed-line' before the audience had finished laughing. The result of his untimely intervention was that the audience was forced to stop laughing, in order to start listening to the beginning of the next joke. The star's moment of glory was lost. In theatrical terms, the action of speaking a new line, thus causing the audience to stop enjoying the last joke in order to listen to the next one is called 'treading on the laugh'. Just how serious a transgression of the unwritten rules of show business 'treading on the laugh' is considered to be by some professional comedians, was made clear to the inexperienced entertainer, when the star apparently expressed his dissatisfaction – with a 'punch-line' of a different kind – after the show.

When considering the use of silence, the clinical nurse supervisor may gain much from this hard-won experience. If the clinical nurse supervisor intervenes too quickly after her supervisee has spoken, she may place the supervisee in a position of being unable to fully appreciate what is happening to him on an emotional level.

Understanding in clinical supervision owes as much to the potential for the supervisee to feel as for him to talk. There is a danger that the supervisor can lose the important opportunity for the enhancement of understanding in the supervisee, by rushing in to speak immediately after the supervisee stops speaking – thereby denying him the chance to think more, and feel more, about the words spoken. I refer to this inapt and limiting technique – with acknowledgement to the entertainer's experience – as *treading on the silence*.

Clinical nurse supervisors can learn to allow their supervisees a space – perhaps even a pregnant pause – between the words in order that they can both fully appreciate what is happening as a result of what has been said. Although it is unlikely – but not impossible – that anyone will want to laugh, there is the potential for a wide range of other feelings to be engendered in both supervisee and supervisor, which can inform the process of supervision if they can be savoured for at least a short time.

Scenario 1, below, in which a supervisee is explaining about the sudden death of a patient, is an example of what might happen when the clinical nurse supervisor treads on the supervision silence. Scenario 2, which uses a similar situation, offers a simple technique to help supervisors to avoid 'treading on the silence':

Scenario 1: The supervisor treads on the silence

Supervisee: . . . I think a lot of us are upset about it really. There was no warning and none of the clinical team really expected it to happen as and when it did. Some of the team also think that perhaps we could have done more to be prepared for the death, if not actually prevent it. [*Looks thoughtful.*]

Supervisor: [*without pausing*] What more could you have done to be prepared?

Supervisee: I didn't say that I was unprepared. Why did you say that? Do *you* think that I was unprepared?

Supervisor: Oh . . . no, not really. That's not what I was suggesting [*awkward pause*] Were you unprepared for it?

Supervisee: No. I'm a professional.

Supervisor: I see. Ermm . . . on another matter . . . you were telling me earlier about the excellent work you did with the nursing students . . .

Scenario 2: The supervisor creates new understanding for her supervisee

Supervisee: . . . I think a lot of us are upset about it really. There was no warning and none of the clinical team really expected it to happen as and when it did. Some of the team also think that perhaps we could have done more to be prepared for the death, if not actually prevent it. [*Looks thoughtful.*]

Supervisor: [*remains silent for 5 seconds*]. I was wondering how you were feeling about it, just now. [*Falls silent.*]

Supervisee: Well, concerned naturally. It's difficult to think that as professionals we might not always get it right.

Supervisor: [*nods and stays silent for 5 seconds.*] Ummm . . . is that what you think might have happened in this case?

Supervisee: I'm not sure.

Supervisor: We could sit quietly for few moments and think about it. [*Falls silent.*]

Supervisee: [*two minutes later*] Now that you've given me some time to reflect I think that we did all we could, actually. But, it's an important lesson to learn that as nurses, there may always be new precautions that we can take and new situations that may arise to challenge us. That we do not always have the answers to everything that might happen.

Supervisor: [*nods and remains silent for 5 seconds*] I see.

Making statements

While the prudent use of questions by the clinical nurse supervisor can assist the promotion of important clinical material necessary to aid the supervisee's reflection on his nursing practice, the continual use of such a limited and limiting device can have potentially detrimental effects on the supervision relationship.

Clinical nurse supervisors wishing to promote imaginative reflection on practice, should think carefully about using questions as their main intervention style. The constant use of questions can quickly lead to the clinical supervisor adopting the persona of a professional inquisitor, with the result that her supervisee can feel as if he is sitting under a bright spot-lamp, compelled to give prompt and correct answers to any and all questions thrown at him.

Meta-communication and meta-questions

Hobson states that: 'embodied in a message is some information about *how* a communication should be received – what sort of message it is' (1985: 193). This information is passed to the receiver of the message through the use of 'cues'. The sender of the message may raise his voice to show that he is angry, move closer to the receiver to demonstrate affection, roll up his sleeves to show that he his considering violence or widen his eyes to express shock and surprise. Whatever cues are used, Hobson sees these actions as a secondary form of message-sending, which he calls 'meta-communication'. It is the underlying message that characterises the primary communication and gives it meaningfulness. Meta-communication is not about *what you say* but rather *how you say it*.

Taking Hobson's work a stage further, I use the term *meta-question* to describe discrete verbal interactions, rather than complete messages. Meta-questions have the double advantage of being very simple devices for the supervisor to accomplish with a little practice, and also interventions that are open to contradiction. Through the use of meta-questions the supervisor adopts a negotiating style that implies that she is not the 'fount of all knowledge' and that the supervisee's perception of the experience is paramount. A supervisee can become tired, very quickly, when faced with a barrage of questions about his work. A supervision session that starts to feel more like a television quiz will soon lose its appeal. A far more amenable approach is for the supervisor to enter into a conversation with her supervisee. She can do this by offering her professional opinions in the form of personal statements, which the supervisee can disagree with, if he wishes. Meta-questions not only have the effect of making questions more 'conversational', they can also reduce the immobilising effects of direct questions. If for example, the supervisor wanted to test out her view about how the supervisee was feeling following a disagreement with a colleague she might do so by using one of at least three different sentences:

(a) 'Are you angry?'
(b) 'You are obviously angry about this, aren't you?'
(c) 'It seems to me that it is the sort of situation that could make you feel angry.'

Sentence (a) is a direct question that is likely to have the effect of putting the supervisee firmly on the spot and feeling that he needs to find an answer quickly. It is also a 'closed question' which can mean that, even if he is in a position to answer it honestly, his response may be limited to a simple 'yes' or 'no' and therefore will not be conducive to a continuing *reflective conversation*. Sentence (b), while not a strictly a question, is certainly a very bold statement – with the persuasive and aggressive quality of a leading question. This style of statement is less conducive to honest reflection than even the closed question in (a), chiefly because its structure may make it extremely difficult for the supervisee to feel that he can disagree. Sentence (c) contains many of the key characteristics of the *meta-question*.

The components of meta-questions

'Meta-question' not only describes a sentence that has been *changed* from a question into a statement, but also indicates sentences that contains certain key words that encourage conversational movement. I offer, below, my suggestions for four sub-categories of the meta-question itself, and their various purposes.

OWNERS

The clinical nurse supervisor is not a 'fount of all knowledge', nor is she speaking officially on behalf of all nurses and all clinical nurse supervisors – and it is imperative that she constantly strives not to imply otherwise to her supervisee. Accordingly, whatever she wishes to say should be couched in terms that suggest she recognises that what she is saying is, primarily, her own opinion. The supervisee must ultimately be the judge of whether something concerning himself is correct or open to change. When the supervisor uses words such as 'I' , 'my' or 'me' in a meta-question, they operate as 'owners' and indicate that the supervisee is being offered a personal opinion which is open to negotiation and, if necessary, change.

NEGOTIATORS

A 'negotiator' can be used in conjunction with an 'owner' to strengthen the emphasis on the *changeable* quality of the personal opinion being offered in the meta-question. The supervisor is offering her view, together with the implicit suggestion that it can be contradicted or altered, if necessary, and as required, by the supervisee. Commonly used 'negotiators' are such words as: 'perhaps', 'maybe', 'view', 'opinion', 'change', 'disagree', and such phrases as: 'is it possible that . . .', 'to my mind' and 'it seems to me . . .'.

GENERALISATIONS

When a delicate or potentially sensitive clinical issue is being discussed, the supervisor may wish to tread carefully when first broaching the subject. Words such as: 'type' 'kind' and 'sort' can be used to suggest that the supervisor is (a) not necessarily referring to the situation currently being discussed, and (b) nor is she referring to it in isolation of other similar situations. This allows for (i) contradiction and negotiation by the supervisee and (ii) may offer the supervisor a useful opening to discuss the supervisee's difficulties or concerns with similar clinical situations either specifically or in a general sense.

MUTABLES

Words such as 'could', 'may' and 'might' are what I refer to as mutables. They allow the supervisee to agree with the premise in a general sense, if not a specific one. The use of a 'mutable' within a meta-question could be seen as an open invitation from the supervisor for the supervisee to contradict or alter the basic premise of the statement. Supervisors should be careful to avoid the use of immutable words such as 'did' or 'must', which do not offer room for contradiction, movement and change by the supervisee.

EXPRESSION SPECIFIERS

In the example of a meta-question below, the word 'feel' is used before the word 'angry', to specify exactly the manner in which the supervisee's anger might have been expressed. It could have been replaced with 'shouted angrily' or 'thrown something in anger' or 'had angry thoughts'. I call all such phrases 'expression specifiers'. Had the supervisor omitted the word 'feel', the supervisee could agree with the notion of anger without having to agree with the suggestion about its specific mode of expression.

Think about . . . the components of meta-questions

Negotiators
Use of 'seems' allows for contradiction and change by supervisee.

Owners
Use of 'me' (or 'I') shows that the supervisor is offering a personal opinion.

'It seems to me that it is the type of situation that could make you feel angry.'

Generalisations
Words such as: 'type', 'kind' and 'sort' are used to suggest that the supervisor is (a) not necessarily referring to the situation currently being discussed, and (b) nor is she referring to it in isolation of other similar situations. This allows for (a) contradiction by the supervisee and (b) a useful opening to discuss difficulties with similar situations.

Mutables
Words such as 'could', 'may' and 'might' are what I refer to as *mutables*. They allow the supervisee to agree with the premise in a general sense, if not a specific one. The supervisor is careful to avoid the use of *immutable* words such as 'did' or 'must', which do not offer room for contradiction, movement and change by the supervisee.

Expression specifiers
In this example of a meta-question, the word *feel* is used before the word 'angry', to specify exactly the manner in which the supervisee's anger might have been expressed. It could have been replaced with 'shouted angrily' or 'thrown something in anger' or 'had angry thoughts'. I call all such phrases '*expression specifiers*'. Had the supervisor omitted the word 'feel', the supervisee could agree with the notion of anger without having to agree with the suggestion about its specific mode of expression.

With reference to the example above, change the following sentences into *meta-questions* that contain characteristics of negotiation, ownership, generalisations, mutables and expression specifiers.

1 You obviously find record-keeping tiresome and boring.
2 Tell me all about it.
3 Why are you smiling?
4 You disagree frequently with your colleagues, don't you?
5 Why are you always late for your shift?

Specific statements for specific situations

Learning how to achieve mutual understanding of the super-visee's experiences and behaviour should be considered a primary concern for the clinical nurse supervisor. In order to do this more effectively, the supervisor can employ a variety of types of statements that have specific actions and tasks that, if used carefully, can be effective in allowing the supervisor to focus her interventions and bring about wider and clearer understanding of the supervisee's work and her feelings about it.

Lieberman and Cobb (1987b) have described broad categories of statements that can be used in interview situations, by doctors and other health professionals, which are themselves based to some extent on the work of Ivey and Simek-Downing (1980) and Heron (1975). A key factor for Lieberman and Cobb, in devising the statement categories, is that the user can control the level of 'intent' – what it is they are trying to do or convey by their statement at any given time – in the interview situation. They state that this concern for specific intention 'distinguishes a professional interview from an ordinary conversation' (1987b: 594).

Lieberman and Cobb explain that a problem with trainee inter-viewers is that, without guidance, they can sometimes make the mistake when starting discussions of intimidating the inter-viewee with in-depth, confronting statements or similarly unsuit-able interventions rather than using welcoming introductory statements. Separating statements into broad categories of 'intent' offers the user more control over what they say and when they say it. I have adapted Lieberman and Cobb's statement 'categories' to the purposes of clinical supervision for nurses, and have tabled them, below, with a description of how they can best be used to the supervisee's advantage.

Giving and receiving feedback in clinical supervision

I see the process of giving feedback as the stock-in-trade of the clinical nurse supervisor. Alongside being listened to and sup-ported, receiving feedback is a major reason that nurses give for choosing to meet with clinical supervisors. Understanding the general principles of the process, in an attempt to ensure that the feedback we offer is delivered in the most accurate, least threat-ening and facilitative manner possible, should be an important goal for those of us involved in the business of offering our thoughts to others.

Table 4.2 *Various types of statements for use by clinical supervisors*

Type of statement	Typical supervision intention	Typical supervision situation	Examples	Comments
Introductory	Setting the scene. Who (and what) you are. How much time you have available. What you intend to do with the supervisee during that time.	First clinical supervision meeting. Limited (part) use in subsequent supervision sessions: (i) in order to clarify any outstanding issues from the previous session (ii) to invite the supervisee to begin with a 'review' of the previous session.	'Hello I'm Sarah, you must be Kevin. We have three quarters of an hour – going by that clock on the wall, to talk about your clinical nursing work.' 'Are there any particular issues that you would like to start with Kevin?' 'To begin this session, is there anything you would like to raise from the last time we met, Kevin?'	Many supervisors like to use a similar form of statement at the end of each supervision session to offer a review of the session and to invite the supervisee to bring back any outstanding or new material to the next session. E.g. 'Our time is up for this session and we have covered much ground today, Kevin, including a discussion of __ and __. I would be happy for us to continue with any or all of these issues next time, if you would like to raise them again.'
Reassuring	To confirm appropriateness of supervisee's input.	Whenever the supervisee may be concerned that his intended material is unsuitable or inappropriate (such as	'That you have become distressed by Mr Brown's death sounds, to me, like something that we might usefully discuss in supervision.'	A problem with the over-use of 'reassuring' statements is that the supervisee can learn to give the supervisor what he thinks she wants and to avoid the issues that he thinks she may not approve.

continued overleaf

Table 4.2 *continued*

Type of statement	Typical supervision intention	Typical supervision situation	Examples	Comments
		with potentially emotive material) and the supervisor feels – after consideration – that it is suitable for discussion in supervision.	'I think that it is perfectly understandable that you feel angry about what you feel has happened to you.'	'Reassuring' statements must be used sparingly in order to be effective and to avoid the supervisee becoming dependent upon, and directed by, the supervisor's view on what may be appropriate or inappropriate input. Ultimately, the supervisee should be free to choose what he will or will not say in the supervision session.
		Often combined with, or substituted for, 'encouraging' statements.		
Encouraging	To enable the supervisee to continue speaking or to elucidate a particular issue.	Whenever the supervisor feels that further information would be enlightening and/or informative.	'Go on.' 'I see.'	Certain 'encouraging' statements can be very similar in style to other categories such as 'prompting' statements. The only criteria in such cases should be the supervisor's intent for the statement's use.
		Frequently used when the supervisee's presentation flow slows down or dries up and the supervisor requires more information.	'Can you say a bit more about what happened after she did that . . .?' 'You were saying that you were late coming on duty . . . [*pause*]' 'You took the syringe and . . . [*pause*]'	Once the supervisor is clear on how she intends the statement to be used, this will then often be signalled to the supervisee through the use of tone of voice and body language.

| **Summarising** | To offer a précis of what the supervisee has said. Offering confirmation that the supervisor has been listening and has understood the gist of the supervisee's input/comments. | Often used at a break in the supervisee's speech, especially if a large amount of material has been presented and/or the supervisee has been speaking for more than a few minutes. | 'Well, as I understand it, the day started well, following the phone call to say that you had been selected for the course, but then things started to go wrong when the new patient was admitted . . . [*pause*] is that about right, so far?' | A useful purpose of 'summarising' statements is that it allows the supervisor to be clear about whether she has fully grasped the gist of the supervisee's comments.

It also offers a period of 'thinking time', in which the supervisor, while recapping the supervisee's input, can collect her thoughts about the issues being raised.

Summarising after the supervisee has raised more than one issue can allow the supervisor an opportunity to segregate different issues and, with the supervisee's co-operation, separate the issues into discrete sections, in order that they can be worked on individually or by making links that connect them together. |
| **Clarifying/ checking** | The supervisor asks for further information to ensure that she has fully understood certain facts that the supervisee has previously offered. | Should be used whenever something in the supervisee's presentation is unclear.

Also used whenever the supervisor needs to | 'Could you just remind me how long you have been a staff nurse on the ITU?'

'I have forgotten the name of the conference | Clinical nurse supervisors, no matter how experienced, will at some point need to seek clarification from the supervisee.

This may be because she has misheard some detail of information |

continued overleaf

Table 4.2 continued

Type of statement	Typical supervision intention	Typical supervision situation	Examples	Comments
	The supervisor confirms that what she thinks she has understood is, in fact, a correct version of events.	confirm specific facts/figures or other details of the supervisee's presentation.	that you were attending just after we met last time?'	or has become distracted during the supervisee's presentation, and realises that she has missed vital facts and figures, or even that she has completely lost 'track' of what is being discussed.
			'I'm sorry, but I seem to have missed part of what you were saying about ____. Could you please just remind me of it.'	Supervisors must resist the temptation to bluff their way through the supervisee's presentation.
			'Am I right in thinking that you have been on the ITU for three years now?'	It is the mark of a skilled and professional clinical nurse supervisor that she is able to stop the discussion in order to clarify or check a point, in order that she is clear to offer the accurate feedback from that point onwards, or even to recap previous feedback.
Focusing	The supervisor selects specific aspects of the supervisee's discussion to discuss in more detail.	Used whenever the supervisor wishes to concentrate on a specific aspect that has been	'I would like stay focused on what you were you saying about ____ for a bit longer.'	The supervisor may choose to focus on one aspect of the supervisee's comments, especially if more than one issue is raised at one time.

	mixed together with other information, in a long, complex and/or detailed presentation.	'Perhaps you could say more about ___.'	Focusing can be used effectively after the supervisor has ascertained the specific issues through the use of 'summarising' statements. 'Focusing' statements can be used in a broad sense such as: 'I would like to hear more about your work on the ITU.' Or very specifically: 'I would like to hear more about your first day on the ITU' or even more specifically: 'I would like to hear more about what happened with Mr Jones on your first day on ITU.' Or extremely specifically: I would like to hear more about why you said you felt 'shattered' after meeting Mr Jones on your first day on ITU.'
Prompting	The supervisor uses devices to encourage the supervisee to continue speaking – or to say more – about a specific issue.	'You were telling me about ___.'	A useful device for 'prompting' statements is the 'unfinished sentence'. The supervisor begins a sentence but stops speaking towards the end of the sentence. If used skilfully, the supervisee will pick up the sentence and add his own word(s) to it to finish it more accurately than the supervisor would
	Used whenever the supervisee seems 'stuck' in his presentation and the supervisor wishes to hear more on the same subject or issue.	'. . . You were in the office and then . . . [pause]'	
	Can be substituted with 'encouraging' statements. however,	*Supervisee*: I remember that it happened just after I had taken	

continued overleaf

Table 4.2　continued

Type of statement	Typical supervision intention	Typical supervision situation	Examples	Comments
		'prompting' statements are often used in a more specific and detailed manner.	Mr Jones' Blood Pressure. *Supervisor:* I see . . . you had just taken Mr Jones' blood pressure and . . . [*pause*]	have been able to do, if she finished it herself: *Supervisor:* I was just thinking that it is the sort of situation that could make you feel a bit . . . [*pause*] *Supervisee:* . . . de-skilled, yes. Another form of 'prompting' statement is for the supervisor to repeat the last sentence or part of the last sentence spoken by the supervisee. It should be noted that all techniques and particularly stylised forms of statements such as the prompting statement types described above, can, at best, become ineffective and, at worst, cause the supervisor to appear foolish if over-used.

| Empathic | The supervisor tries to indicate that she has some sense of how the supervisee is feeling or reacting in regard to the issue being discussed. | Can be used when the supervisor senses that the supervisee may feel alone in his concerns or in some way 'isolated' by his presentation. | 'It would not be right for me to suggest that I know *exactly* how it must have been for you, but perhaps you can help me to get a clearer understanding of the situation.'

'It seems to me that you could have been left feeling — by that.'

'An incident like that is the sort of thing that can make nurses feel ___. I wonder if that applies to you, too?'

'This does seem to me, to be quite difficult for you.' | To be effective, 'empathic' statements of the 'I guess you might be having feelings about this' type require the supervisor to be either reasonably accurate in his assumption of how the supervisee may be feeling and/or should be couched in such terms as to allow the supervisee to change the suggested 'feeling' to one that fits his situation more accurately.

Supervisors (and health professionals generally) should always avoid making statements of the: 'I know how you must be feeling variety. Such statements are likely to be grossly inaccurate, because knowing how someone feels even about a situation that the speaker may have experienced is virtually impossible due to the peculiarities of human perception. They can also be considered insulting or offensive to the listener, for similar reasons. |

continued overleaf

Table 4.2 *continued*

Type of statement	Typical supervision intention	Typical supervision situation	Examples	Comments
Self-revelatory	The supervisor makes a personal statement – usually based on her nursing work – to inform or otherwise facilitate the supervisee in the presentation of his clinical material.	Can be used in a similar way to 'empathic' statements (above). When used with certain models of supervision can be used to allow the supervisor to offer new insights on the supervisee's material (see Chapter 6).	'My first experience of ITU was daunting to begin with, until I began to settle into the work and gain my confidence.' 'I remember trying to tell my supervisor about the time a patient died. I tried to be so professional about it, thinking that she would disapprove of me showing my true feelings.'	If used carefully and sparingly, self-disclosure by the clinical nurse supervisor can be a powerful way to encourage, reassure and even prompt the supervisor. It must be remembered however, that the clinical supervision is not a forum for the supervisor to relive her clinical memoirs or to 'hold court' over her subjects. If the supervisor is to use self-revelation, she must ensure that it is used briefly and carefully and always in the best interests of the supervisee, who should constantly remain the focal-point of the supervision session.

There are many different ways to tell someone how we feel about the things that they have said and done. Some will prefer the direct, no-punches-pulled 'I-call-a-spade-a-bloody-shovel' approach, perhaps seeing it as the most open and honest method of saying how we feel about a certain issue. It certainly has its advantages. The receiver of the feedback will be left in no doubt as to how we feel.

Others opt for the more reflective position, picking up on the things that people say without direct comment of their own. At its extreme this can cause the speaker to feel that she is being constantly quizzed – in a huge echo chamber, as in the following exchange:

> *First nurse*: I was really furious and so I told him that if I didn't get an apology quickly I would see his boss and complain!
> *Second nurse*: You certainly were really furious! What did he say to that?
> *First nurse*: He just looked blankly at me and I poked him with my brolly. It's got a sharp point.
> *Second nurse*: That brolly certainly has got a very sharp point, you poked me with it once, I can vouch for its sharpness. So, what happened next?

Think about . . . the quality of supervision feedback

Read the following extracts from clinical supervision and put yourself in the position of the supervisee hearing the supervisor's feedback. Try to answer the questions for each extract before moving on to the next section.

EXTRACT 1

> *Supervisee*: I'm concerned about what happened last Tuesday. I overslept and arrived on the ward nearly two hours late. Another nurse was allocated my patients in addition to her own and she was very stressed and angry with me when I finally turned up.
> *Supervisor 1*: I am not surprised. You are the world's most unreliable nurse.

1 Summarise the general nature of the feedback.
2 Describe how it might feel to receive these comments.
3 Do you consider the feedback to be fair, reasonable and balanced?
4 What would you expect to be your most likely response to this feedback?

EXTRACT 2

> *Supervisee*: I'm concerned about what happened last Tuesday. I overslept and arrived on the ward nearly two hours late. Another nurse was allocated my patients in addition to her own and she was very stressed and angry with me when I finally turned up.

> *Supervisor 2*: Try not to worry about it. We all make mistakes from
> time to time and I'm sure the other nurse was over-reacting to being
> asked to take on extra work. I advise you forget all about it and
> carry on as if nothing has happened.
>
> 1 Summarise the general nature of the feedback.
> 2 Do you consider the feedback to be fair, reasonable and balanced?
> 3 What would be your response to this feedback?

Had you been the hapless supervisee on the receiving end of
Supervisor 1, you may well wish that you had never mentioned the
situation at all. The likelihood of you wanting to raise concerns
about your own professional conduct to that supervisor ever again,
could also be fairly slim! The supervisor's response is subjective,
critical, unbalanced, unfair and it could very well leave the supervisee feeling discouraged from attending supervision again.

A major problem with the feedback from Supervisor 2 above, is
that although the supervisee may not want to run screaming from
the room vowing never to return, as might happen in the first
scenario, the supervision comments have the potential to be just as
unhelpful as those of Supervisor 1.

What's the point of feedback?
- Feedback helps the receiver to become more aware of what
  they do and how they do it.
- Receiving feedback gives the supervisee an opportunity to
  change and modify their actions in order to become more
  effective and responsible nurses.
- In order to be constructive, feedback needs to be offered in a
  concerned and supportive manner.
- In order that the supervisee can grow professionally, feedback
  may need to include – over time – both positive and negative
  observations.

CORBS and the art of giving feedback
We all develop our styles of feedback over time and there is no
one single approach that is necessarily better or worse than any
other. The most appropriate style is likely to be one that is balanced
and thoughtful, given the supervisee's comments, behaviour and
emotional state at the time. There are some useful guidelines for
giving and receiving feedback, which can be readily applied to

clinical supervision which are often explained by the acronym CORBS.

Make sure your feedback fits the CORBS rule
- **C** is for supervision feedback that is clear
- **O** is for supervision feedback that is owned
- **R** is for supervision feedback that is regular
- **B** is for supervision feedback that is balanced
- **S** is for supervision feedback that is specific

KISS to make sure your feedback is clear
Clear clinical supervision feedback is concerned with saying what you mean and meaning what you say. If what you say is precise – and concise – there will be less room for doubt and confusion in the mind of the supervisee. Giving supervision feedback that is clear is a skill that will take practice to perfect.

For a guideline to help in the delivery of clear supervision feedback follow the rule of KISS – *Keep It Simple, Stupid!* Banish long words and long sentences from your supervision sessions. Get short and simple. Be concise and be clear. Remember that convoluted is complicated and complicated is confusing. The supervisee is not the only person likely to become confused, either!

A friend of mine jokes that he will never use one word when six or seven will do. Forget all about that maxim during clinical supervision. Trying to become too clever with words can leave you appearing dogmatic, pompous and – worst of all – boring. There is much more chance of losing your train of thought, and missing the point, by setting off on a long and ultimately aimless ramble. A vicious circle can ensue as you become increasingly anxious about not making your point. You start to falter and hesitate and your message becomes indecipherable.

To ensure that you make and maintain a reputation for the clearest clinical supervision feedback remember that brevity is best and simple is superior.

Owned up!
What you have to say as a clinical supervisor may be interesting and even, on rare occasions, important to others, but it is not the ultimate truth. It is essential that your supervisee understands this too as, for some, there will be a tendency to want to invest supervisors with an omnipotence that they do not deserve and

certainly cannot live up to. Being a clinical supervisor for nurses puts you in a very awkward position. People will really start to listen to what you will say to them! As a group, supervisees who are starting out will tend to treat the things said to them by experienced (or senior) nurses very seriously indeed. Throw-away remarks made half-jokingly in the staff room during tea-break may be instantly forgotten by all those within ear-shot if you are in I'm-just-another-member-of-the-ward-team mode. It can be quite a shock to the system to discover those very same unimportant asides being widely related throughout the organisation as the-thoughts-of-supervisor-Smith by your new – and very proud – supervisee!

Taking care of what you say to supervisees is an extremely important task of clinical supervision for nurses. At times, it can seem like everything you are about to say needs to be put through some sort of mental clearing house for double-checking. I suggest that, at least to begin with, that is exactly how it should be. Think about what you are about to say. Think again – is it appropriate? Then say it.

A nurse widely regarded by her colleagues as a 'know-all', told me that she had been accused of being dogmatic. 'They have got it all wrong', she protested indignantly, 'how can I possibly be dogmatic, when dogmatic means arrogantly believing that you are right about an issue without evidence or proof.' She paused for breath and I smiled at her and waited expectantly for further proof that this most dogmatic of dogmatists had – in fact – finally seen the light. The smile was quickly wiped from my lips as she went blindly on: 'Surely I could only be thought of as dogmatic if I believed myself to be right when I am, in fact wrong?' I had to agree with this irrefutable statement and nodded politely. 'Well, there you are then. How can I possibly be dogmatic. I *am* always right about everything that I say!'

My rule for ensuring that clinical supervision feedback is owned is: think before you speak and then speak only what you think. Prefacing statements with phrases such as: 'I sometimes find that . . .', 'It seems to me . . .', 'In my view . . .', 'I have an idea that . . .' can help to convey the message that what you are saying is your own (and owned) personal view. Supervisees will find difficult statements, especially about their work and behaviour, much easier to consider and respond to, if they feel that they are being offered a personal opinion – however well informed – and not the last and only word on the subject.

Keep yourself regular

It is important that supervision feedback should not only be given as clearly as possible and from the perspective of the supervisor, but that it should also be offered on a consistently regular basis. If the supervisor leaves long gaps between feedback it might cause the supervisee to move on to another issue before she has commented on the previous one. The supervisee could well be forgiven for thinking that the supervisor has no opinion on the matter (in which case, it is often preferable for the supervisor to simply state this fact than say nothing) or is disinterested in the matter being raised by the supervisee. Try to give feedback as soon as possible after the issue is raised, and at least, early enough for the supervisee to practically respond to suggestions, if necessary.

A more difficult, but equally important aspect of regular supervision feedback involves the supervisor monitoring her level of input over a period of several sessions or more. It would be ludicrous to suggest that supervisors attempt to regulate their supervision feedback to guarantee that each utterance matches the last in terms of quality, length or in any other way. However, it is sensible for supervisors to mentally check that the supervisee is not confused by one clinical supervision session consisting of virtually no feedback and the next involving the supervisor making long speeches.

Check that it balances

If supervision feedback is required to be clear, owned and regular, it follows that it should also be perceived by the supervisee as being properly balanced. As with the process of monitoring the regularity of the feedback, the supervisor should try, over time, to maintain a balanced blend of comment, instruction, advice and facilitated reflection, depending, of course on the needs of the supervisee.

At the very least, when offering comment and instruction, the supervisor should try to ensure – over time and not necessarily during the same supervision session – that she provides a reasonably balanced amount of positive and negative feedback, in a general sense. If the supervisor provides only one kind of feedback it is likely that the supervisee will come to – justifiably – suspect that the supervisor's view of him is distorted. Lots of positive feedback at the beginning of a course of clinical supervision may encourage the supervisee to feel that he or she has made the right decision in choosing to be supervised. However, supervisees are likely to quickly become disheartened if the supervisor continues to confer upon them nothing but plaudits several weeks into the supervision period.

It is important that the supervisee is encouraged to grow and develop throughout the supervision process. Positive and encouraging feedback must therefore be balanced with comments and instruction that allow him to revisit and rethink erroneous thoughts and actions in a way that can bring about a more workable solution for all those concerned. The supervisor should monitor her feedback to ensure that encouragingly positive comments are balanced over time with growth-enhancing ones and that neither sort dominates the sessions. This situation would sooner-or-later result in the supervisee becoming dissatisfied with, and ultimately losing faith in his supervisor.

'You talkin' to me?' – be specific!

Imagine that two friends have just returned from an evening at the cinema, and are now eating the take-away they bought from the drive-through at the local fast food restaurant. The conversation goes a bit like this:

> *Friend 1*: The film was good wasn't it? A real tear-jerker. I'm glad I brought extra tissues, I love crying at the cinema – it's good for the appetite even though I am on a diet.
>
> *Friend 2*: Yes that was a real tear-jerker, I nearly filled my pop corn bucket. Anyway, let's eat, I'm starving!
>
> *Friend 1*: There are so many people who can't cry though, even if they wanted to, and I think it's a shame. Perhaps they're embarrassed or something.
>
> *Friend 2*: More nuggets or fries? I ordered extra large portions.
>
> *Friend 1*: [*taking more nuggets and a handful of fries*] I mean; it's nothing to be ashamed of but lots of people *say* they've cried and yet they haven't really. I mean, if they can't cry it's OK, but at least they should not try to pretend they have! Oh, you might want these tissues back, you didn't use all of them.
>
> *Friend 2*: The other thing that is so annoying is when people say that they are dieting but carry on eating as normal. Why can't they just say that they don't want to be bothered!
>
> *Friend 1*: Would you like some of my fries, I've got lots?
>
> *Both together*: Erm . . . are you trying to tell me something?

Generalised feedback is hard to learn from and easy to ignore. Temper what you say by all means, there is little point in being unnecessarily rude or bruisingly blunt for its own sake. If you want to tell a supervisee something about his work – good or not so good – make sure that he knows that you are talking about him specifically. It will be easier for him to respond and should have the added advantage of ensuring that you are certain of what you want to say – and that you want to say it – before you speak.

Being specific means not just making sure that both supervisor and supervisee know who is being talked about but also what is the issue under discussion. It is not out of the question that a supervisor will want to tell a supervisee that they have induced a certain feeling in them. This may involve expressing positive feelings of pleasure and satisfaction or not-so-positive ones.

Whatever you need to tell your supervisee about how you are feeling should be done in a way that specifically links the supervisor's feeling or viewpoint with an action or behaviour belonging to the supervisee. This avoids what I call the trap of generalisation in which the supervisor becomes caught up in allowing the supervisee to believe that everything that he does is pleasing or – conversely – that he is and will remain constantly irritating, annoying or incompetent, no matter what he does now or will do in the future.

In the dialogue below, the supervisor is attempting to convey a feeling she has about the supervisee emanating from a problem with his work and which could well be shared by his colleagues. Unfortunately, the supervisor's wide generalisation of her feelings traps the supervisee into making an unnecessary but, under the circumstances, understandable response.

> *Supervisor 1*: You can be very irritating at times!
> *Supervisee*: As you feel that way about me, perhaps I should find another supervisor!

In the following dialogue extract, the supervisor has avoided the trap of generalisation by linking her feelings directly to a behaviour belonging to the supervisee.

> *Supervisor 2*: I feel irritated when you tell me that you, once again, forgot to make a record of the treatment in Mr Brown's case notes until the next day. Perhaps I'm not alone in feeling like that, too.
> *Supervisee*: As you feel that way, I can see that my colleagues could feel even more strongly about it. I'll be a lot more careful to record the treatment immediately from now on.

Had you been the hapless supervisee on the receiving end of Supervisor 1, you may well wish that you had never mentioned the situation at all. The likelihood of you wanting to raise concerns about your own professional conduct to that supervisor ever again, could also be fairly slim! The supervisor's response is subjective, critical, unbalanced, unfair and it could very well leave the supervisee feeling discouraged from attending supervision again.

A major problem with the feedback from Supervisor 2 above, is that although the supervisee may not want to run screaming from the room vowing never to return, as might happen in the first scenario, the supervision comments have the potential to be just as unhelpful as those of Supervisor 1.

By making the feedback specific the supervisor has produced a completely different response in the supervisee, who no longer feels not-good-enough for the supervisor in a very general and all-encompassing way, but can associate the irritation with a specific – and probably isolated – problem in his work. His response is considered and much less defensive. He even volunteers the information that his colleagues are aggrieved with him – something he may have suspected anyway. Best of all, he offers to address the situation and the supervision relationship continues, undamaged.

The focus of clinical supervision feedback
The focus of feedback in clinical supervision should always be on:

- The behaviour of the supervisee rather than the person.
  What he does not who we imagine him to be.
  Use adverbs that relate to actions rather than adjectives which relate to qualities.
- Observations rather than inferences.
  What was actually said and done, rather than the supervisor's assumptions of why it occurred.
- Description rather than judgement.
- Specifics rather than generalisations.
- Sharing ideas and information rather than giving advice.
- Personal ownership of ideas rather than sweeping statements.
- The amount of information the supervisee can use rather than the amount the supervisor would like to give.

Helping the supervisee to make the most of feedback
Clinical supervisors should consider offering the following guidelines to supervisees in order that you can both work together to ensure high quality, growth enhancing supervision feedback.

LISTEN TO THE FEEDBACK RECEIVED FROM YOUR SUPERVISOR WITHOUT JUDGING IT
Try not to jump to a defensive response, even though your initial feelings may be of hurt or anger. Give yourself to time to mull

over in your head what has been said to you and to consider its relevance and value to you. Sometimes it can be helpful to take the feedback 'away' from the supervision session, in your head to consider at a distance.

IF YOUR SUPERVISOR DOES NOT OFFER YOU FEEDBACK THAT IS CORBS –
ASK FOR IT!
Try using or adapting such phrases as:

'When you used the word ___ was I right to think you were referring to . . .'
'Is that your own opinion or the general view?'
'Before we move on, can you say something about the problem I had with . . .'
'Can I ask how you felt about that really good/awful thing that happened last week?'
'You seem to be implying that I am clever/lazy/stupid/caring. Is that feeling connected to something that I specifically did/ said or do you think that is how I seem generally?'

TRY NOT TO COMPULSIVELY AND AUTOMATICALLY EXPLAIN YOUR
ACTIONS
Supervisees should be aware that what they do is not necessarily wrong or inappropriate, even when it is commented upon by their clinical supervisors. Sometimes, it may be the case that as a supervisee you will want to redress an action. At other times the supervisor may be offering you an alternative view of a situation or course of action, which will, in itself, not constitute a criticism and therefore does not demand an explanation of your original action.

If you habitually explain your actions, then there is an inherent danger of good work being explained away, as if it were flawed and undesirable – which will be detrimental to positive professional development.

TRY TO HEAR THE SUPERVISOR'S FEEDBACK AS HER PERSONAL OPINION
OF YOUR WORK
If the supervisor's feedback appears to be either very positive or critical, do not immediately assume that the supervisor is speaking about you on behalf of everyone in the department, the organisation or the nursing profession in general. Supervisors may have their opinions but they are not the keepers of the

ultimate truth about you. Listen to your supervisor's comments with this maxim in mind. Sometimes it is helpful to hear the supervision feedback, say 'thank you' and make a silent appraisal of its value and appropriateness.

ASK FOR FEEDBACK THAT YOU WOULD LIKE ON SPECIFIC AREAS OF YOUR WORK

Try not to assume that the supervisor will necessarily cover all of the work that you are involved with in any given session. If you wish to hear about how the supervisor viewed your handling of a particular situation or your progress generally in a specific area of your professional development, ask for it.

In order to obtain a response that you will find considered and satisfactory, warn the supervisor, in advance, of your desire to hear her views on a given subject. Try mentioning that you have not discussed matter 'x' for a few weeks – perhaps because you have both been busy with situations 'y' and 'z' – and ask if, at the next meeting, the supervisor would consider giving you her views on the issue. If you do this at the beginning of a clinical supervision session, your supervisor might agree to spend some time discussing it towards the end of that meeting, if she had not planned to raise it.

5
The First Supervision Session – and Getting Beyond It!

Key issues in this chapter

- The importance of listening skills
- The 'spaces' of supervisory attention
- The value of self-awareness for clinical supervisors
- What to do during the first supervision session
- What the supervisee should expect from the supervisor – and vice-versa
- Making a supervision contract
- The threats of clinical supervision

Shut up and listen – the art of making no noise!

The first clinical supervision session with a new supervisee can be crucial. It will determine how – and if – you are to proceed with the supervision of that nurse and what form that supervision is likely to take. I have chosen to begin this section with an overview of the often much neglected skill of listening because listening to the supervisee is the first thing, last and most valuable thing that clinical nurse supervisors can do. Until supervisors learn to properly *listen* they will never really *hear* what the supervisee has to say. As a consequence, the feedback they offer is likely to be inadequate – perhaps because it will be based more on what they assume – or decide – has been said to them, rather than what the supervisee really wanted to say.

Three aspects of listening
Three main aspects of effective listening can be described as follows:

1 LINGUISTICS

The linguistic aspect of listening is about paying particular attention to the supervisee's spoken language. The supervisor should listen to, and think about, the actual words, phrases and metaphors that the supervisee chooses to convey the particular message he wishes to send, the story that he needs to tell and how he feels about it.

2 PARALINGUISTICS

The paralinguistic aspect of listening involves the supervisor considering all the aspects of her supervisee's speech that are not 'proper' words. It includes: the noises that the supervisee may make as he speaks – coughs, umms, ahhs and ermms – the timing of his words, the volume of his speech – very quiet or very loud – the pitch of his voice, his accent and the tone of his voice. The most telling aspects of paralinguistics may be in how things vary with what is being said, or from session to session, rather than in themselves alone.

3 NON-VERBALS

When the supervisor considers the non-verbal aspects of listening, she will pay close attention to her supervisee's body position and movement, facial expression, use of gestures and his proximity to the supervisor as he speaks. All of these things should be considered in relation to the content of the speech, and, as with paralinguistics, how these things may change over time.

Get SOLER powered – for good listening behaviour

The acronym SOLER can be used to help remember and practise appropriate listening behaviour during a clinical supervision session.

- **S** *Sit squarely* in relation to your supervisee
- **O** Maintain an *open* posture
- **L** *Lean* slightly forward towards the supervisee
- **E** Make regular *eye* contact with the supervisee
- **R** *Relax*

Concentrate on the spaces of supervisory attention

Try to monitor, throughout each supervision session, what you are focused on at any given time. I suggest that there are three key spaces of attention that the supervisor needs to consider in relation to her work with the supervisee and I refer to them as:

1   The space of reality
2   The space of aloneness-togetherness
3   The space of fantasy

1   THE SPACE OF REALITY

The first space of supervisory attention – *the space of reality* – involves a conscious awareness of everything that you, as a clinical supervisor, are doing and the things that your supervisee is doing or saying at any given time. When the supervisor's attention is in the space of reality, it is focused upon:

- The words that are being spoken.
- The body language, posture and gestures that are being displayed.
- The room condition – for example, the need to turn the lights on or take the phone off the hook.
- The time.

2   THE SPACE OF ALONENESS-TOGETHERNESS

This space of attention is concerned with the supervisor having the potential to become 'tuned-in' to what her supervisee is saying, through both introspective and contemplative attention to what is happening 'within' and 'around' her during the supervision. I have used the phrase *Aloneness-togetherness*, originally coined by Hobson (1985), because I feel it best describes the supervisor's simultaneous struggle and opportunity to be alone in her own 'space' and also together with her supervisee in his 'space' at one and the same time. Hobson's phrase, is itself based on the work of the philosopher, Martin Buber (1958) who originally theorised the notion of I-Thou to represent a sense of 'separation with mutality' which will enhance the sense of understanding between two people engaged in a communication. The implicit suggestion here is that, on the one hand, when two people come together, there can be a hidden anxiety about whether the 'gelling' of the individuals will result in loss of their unique identities. On the other hand, there is the implicit danger that, if either partner struggles to remain 'unchanged' in any sense by the 'coming together' with the other person, they can lose a valuable opportunity to gain new insights and understandings.

When the supervisor uses the space of aloneness-togetherness, she allows herself to be drawn into the supervisee's world, without losing her own sense of identity. She can do this in a number of ways, including focusing on her own thoughts and feelings, mental images and gut-feelings which although they may be initially personal in nature, could be connected and related to the themes being discussed by the supervisee.

3   THE SPACE OF FANTASY

The third space of supervisory attention is one I refer to as *the space of fantasy*. This is where nurses may escape to after a hard day on the ward. In this space, we will find the dream holiday that we have not yet enjoyed, the delicious meal that we have not yet eaten and the perfect partner that we have still to meet. Although it may sound tempting, when the clinical nurse supervisor is in this 'space' her supervisory attention is as far away from the supervisee as it could ever get. There is also a strong chance that she may never return from the enticing and wonderful things she will find there – at least not until the end of the supervision session. If supervisors find themselves drifting into this psychological space, they can benefit themselves and their supervisee by considering exactly what may be encouraging them to go there at all. It may be tiredness, general disenchantment with the work or even something about the supervisee himself, that is encouraging the supervisor to 'escape' from the supervision work, but whatever reason is found it should be addressed quickly. The space of fantasy, although it can be enticing, will rarely be a positive influence on a clinical supervision session.

Think about . . . your spaces of attention

Reality
What are your give-away 'boredom-signals'?
How might a colleague become aware that you are losing your
    concentration on his conversation?
Might you:
Fidget or move about more in your seat?
Open and begin to read or write in your diary?
Stop making eye contact and look more at your watch or the door?
'Forget' what either of your were saying?
Insist on making a phone call?

Aloneness–togetherness
What happens when you become more 'in-tune' with another person?
Does your body-language change – do you copy the way that he sits or holds his hands?
Does your spoken language change – do you use words and phrases that may be peculiar to him?
Can you 'see' him, in your 'mind's eye', doing the things that he is talking about?
Do you find yourself 'taking the words out of his mouth' or pre-empting his actions?

Fantasy
What is your favourite 'escapism' fantasy and what is happening around you when you indulge in it?
Is it when:
You are alone – or lonely?
You are in undesirable company?
You feel bored?
You feel sad?
You feel disappointed or unhappy with your circumstances?

Aids to effective listening

There is much that we can do to ensure that as clinical nurse supervisors we listen more effectively to the supervisee. Below is a list of key areas that, if addressed even in part, can result in you being more able to hear clearly what the supervisee wishes you to hear.

- Suspend judgement – do not arrive at any views about the content until the supervisee has finished speaking.
- Concentrate on the SOLER aspects of good listening behaviour until they become second-nature.
- Make sure that the room has comfortable seating, but do not become too relaxed to concentrate properly.
- Make arrangements to avoid extraneous noise and other disturbances and distractions.
- Try not to comment or ask questions until the supervisee has finished speaking.

A valuable consequence of good supervisory listening behaviour will be that the supervisee feels that he is being listened to more intently than ever. This can result in a sort of 'beneficial' circle with the supervisee now taking more care over the things he needs to say – resulting in even more clarity and increased listening behaviour on the part of the supervisor.

Blocks to effective listening

There are a range of factors that can interfere with the clinical nurse supervisor's ability to listen effectively to her supervisee. The vigilant supervisor will try to keep a 'weather-eye' out for these *listening blocks* as they may arise and if it is impossible to avoid them totally, it may be useful to take their possible effect on the supervisor's objectivity into consideration, when considering what the supervisee has to say. They include:

- The supervisor's own personal problems and difficulties.
- The supervisor's own stress and anxiety caused by the work.
- The supervisor's lack of attention to SOLER listening behaviour.
- Making value judgements and misinterpreting what the supervisee is saying.
- The supervisor rehearsing feedback in her head while the supervisee is speaking.
- External noises and distractions.

Personal problems and stress caused by work are serious causes of listening blocks for clinical nurse supervisors. Should such blocks become very persistent, the supervisor may wish to consider discussing her difficulty in staying focused with the supervisee, if not necessarily the specific reasons for this. In extreme cases of listening difficulty – perhaps when the supervisor is in the throes of a personal crisis or outside noise and distractions become excessive – the supervisor may wish to seek external help to alleviate her listening block, either from a colleague or other appropriate professional.

Be aware – be very self-aware!

Clinical nurse supervisors need to develop self-awareness. Not only might it be considered naive – not to say arrogant – for a supervisor to suggest that her responsibility is solely to develop this quality in the supervisee, but such a narrow-minded attitude could result in serious supervisory problems. Some clinical nurse supervisors may balk at the notion of developing their self-awareness. They may even feel insulted by the implicit suggestion that, having reached a senior position in a responsible and highly regarded profession, they have not fully developed as human beings. Well – tough! Swallow your pride and take a good, long look at yourself! I guarantee that the more closely and regularly that you are able to monitor your own thoughts and actions, likes and dislikes, wants and needs and hopes and fears, the better supervisor you will become – and more often than not you will become a better person into the bargain.

Self-awareness is intimately bound up in our relationships with others. As people, we all have differing desires, ambitions, hopes and fears. There is also much that we have in common. If, as supervisors, we have the clearest possible picture of what is happening to ourselves, what we want to do and how we feel about it, then we are better placed to advise our supervisees on their own particular situations.

Gaining self-awareness is not something that we can do quickly or in one fell-swoop. It is a gradual and continuing process of first noticing and then exploring aspects of ourselves that may either be new to us or arise in new situations and settings.

The gaining of self-awareness should always have the con-structive consequence of improving the supervisor's ability to communicate with and better understand her supervisee. Below, is a list of some of the more positive benefits of increased self-awareness that all nurses may wish to consider.

EGO-BOUNDARIES ARE STRENGTHENED
The more we are aware of ourselves as individuals, the less likely it becomes that we fear invasion from someone else's personality. If we are clear about who we are, we can be clear about who we are not. A second benefit of increased ego-boundaries is that issues presented by the supervisee will be less likely to be con-fused with our own. As supervisors this can mean we are of more use to our supervisees because we can avoid becoming swallowed up and lost in their anguish, while remaining concerned.

PERSONAL CHOICE IS INCREASED
To become more aware of ourselves can result in making con-scious, intentional use of our self. We begin to realise how we can act in an honest and congruent way to the full benefit of not only ourselves, but each other. An added bonus of this self-discovery,

can be that we choose to do or not to do something without guilt or self-recrimination.

Some problems of increased self-awareness

In certain cases it is possible that increased self-awareness could have a detrimental effect on the individual. I have outlined below some of the more likely negative effects of self awareness.

INCREASED EGOCENTRICITY

Without reasonable care and self-monitoring the process of increasing our self-awareness could possibly lead to a view that we are the centre of our universe. We may become so caught up with ourselves that we ignore, or worse disregard others in the pursuit of our self-centred ideals. Once embarked on the slippery slope of egocentricity we become self-indulgent, selfish and people more likely to be in need of receiving clinical supervision than capable of providing it.

THE PERFECTION TRAP

It would be a mistake to assume that increased self-awareness inevitably leads to our being better people. This goal, while commendable, is not a natural consequence of knowing ourselves more fully. While we may not become perfect through increased self-regard, it is hoped that we may at least increase our humility, sense of humour and be generally more relaxed about the people that we are.

The first supervision meeting – the establishment phase

The first clinical supervision meeting – or *session*, as I will continue to call it – will often be the one that will determine the course, direction, and to some extent, the outcome of the whole clinical supervision arrangement between a supervisor and her supervisee.

I think of the first clinical supervision session, and perhaps the next two or three, as being part of the *establishment phase* of clinical supervision, because it is during these early sessions that the 'working alliance' between supervisor and supervisee will either be properly established, or permanently destroyed. The first supervision session will be different from probably all of the others that follow it, though, because it will contain specific content, delivered in a specific form and order. The first session will allow both the clinical nurse supervisor and her supervisee to reach a clearly defined understanding of, and agreement on, several important issues, which, in turn, will enhance the potential for establishment of the supervision.

These issues can be split into three sub-groups containing information required by the supervisor; information required by the supervisee; and issues that both supervisor and supervisee need to have come to an agreement on. I will consider each set of information in turn and offer suggestions about how it can best be gathered.

What the supervisor needs to know
At the conclusion of the first clinical supervision session, the supervisor should have gathered enough information to feel reasonably clear in her head that she understands at least something of the following issues:

- Who is the supervisee?
- What does the supervisee want from clinical supervision?
- Why does the supervisee want supervision at this particular point in his career?
- What does the supervisee expect to receive from the supervisor?

Gathering information on the supervisee
If she is to answer these key questions fully, the supervisor will need to seek answers to a range of minor but equally pertinent questions including:

- What is your name?
- Where do you work as a nurse and what do you do there?
- How long have you been in your present post and where else have you worked as a nurse in the last year/two years/ five years (as relevant)?
- What do you think that clinical supervision for nurses is all about?
- What do you want from clinical supervision and how do you think that I can help you to get it?
- Why have you come for clinical supervision at this precise time?

- Have you been supervised previously?
- Why have you chosen me for your clinical supervisor?

The answers that the supervisee gives to the questions will be very helpful in allowing the supervisor to understand:

- This nurse's current experience.
- This nurse's expectations of clinical supervision.
- If this nurse is someone who is seriously intent on being supervised.
- If this nurse understands the process and requirements of clinical supervision.
- If she is appropriately qualified to be the supervisor for this nurse.
- If she is appropriately experienced to be the supervisor for this nurse.

The myth of not questioning the supervisor

It is relevant, at this point, to explode another 'myth' surrounding clinical supervision namely: *supervisees are not supposed to ask supervisors personal questions*. It is not uncommon for both participants involved in this first meeting to assume that only the supervisor is in a position – or worse, is the only one with a right – to ask questions. There may be an implicit assumption that the supervisor is automatically in a 'one-up position' in relation to the supervisee – perhaps due to her more senior professional standing – and, by virtue of this, is the only one allowed to ask questions about professional experience and expertise. Not only would these be erroneous assumptions, but also potentially very dangerous ones that could soon lead to difficulties within the professional relationship. The successful practice of clinical supervision relies much on the quality of the relationship between the supervisor and supervisee for its continued success. In order for this to happen, the supervisee needs to feel able to question, challenge and even contradict his clinical supervisor – within reason – as necessary.

Finding out who the supervisor *is*, in a professional sense, at the outset can go a long way to establishing a balanced supervisory relationship. I would advise all clinical nurse supervisors to encourage their supervisees to ask questions and raise points of debate and challenging issues from the very beginning of the process. It is likely to lead to a much healthier long-term professional relationship.

What the supervisee needs to know

By the end of the first clinical supervision session the supervisee should have asked – and if necessary been encouraged to ask – enough questions to gather relevant information to enable him to be reasonably sure that he understands at least something of the following issues:

- Who is the supervisor?
- What is the supervisor's experience of clinical supervision for nurses?
- What is the supervisor's specialist area(s) of clinical experience and expertise?
- What does the supervisor expect from the supervisee in relation to the clinical supervision?

Gathering information on the supervisor

Pertinent questions that a supervisee might ask of the supervisor at the first clinical supervision session might include:

- What is your name?
- Where do you work as a nurse and what do you do there?
- How long have you been in your present post and where else have you worked as a nurse in the last year/two years/ five years (as relevant)?
- What do you think that clinical supervision for nurses is all about?
- How much experience do you have of supervising nurses?
- Do you prefer any particular model or style of clinical supervision?
- Do you have any specific training in clinical supervision?
- What would be the *minimum* length of time that you could reasonably commit to supervising me?

The answers that the supervisor gives to such questions will be very useful in allowing the supervisee to understand:

- The supervisor's current clinical and supervisory experience.
- This supervisor's style of clinical supervision.
- If the supervisor is someone who is seriously interested in supervising this nurse.

- If the supervisor understands the process and requirements of clinical supervision.
- If she is appropriately qualified to be the supervisor for this nurse.
- The supervisor's level of commitment to supervising this nurse.

The clinical supervision contract

There are issues that both supervisor and supervisee need to have an understanding of, and to have come to an agreement on, before the conclusion of the first clinical supervision session. In essence, these consist of certain ground rules that will make up the clinical supervision contract and form the basis of subsequent sessions. These ground rules refer to essential aspects of the clinical supervision process and delineate certain professional and personal 'boundaries' that both supervisor and supervisee should agree to work within. The more that such boundaries can be adhered to the more successful the clinical supervision will become.

Many practitioners involved in clinical supervision advocate that the key elements of the clinical supervision contract should be written down and signed by both parties at the first session, with copies being held by both supervisor and supervisee for future reference. Ultimately, if time is taken to do this, it can lead to a consolidation of the professional relationship between the clinical nurse supervisor and her supervisee and avoid confusion later on concerning just what was agreed and what was not. Wilkin (1998a), reviewing the literature on contracts for clinical supervision, concludes that although there are: '. . . many suggested formats for a supervision contract . . . the key components seem to be very similar'. Wilkin (in part citing Hawkins and Shohet, 1989) adds that the supervision contract 'basically . . . encourages a reciprocal relationship-orientated approach, whilst outlining the boundaries and individual responsibilities of both supervisor and supervisee' (1998a: 14).

In Figures 5.1 and 5.2 I have replicated a clinical supervision contract used by Rochdale Healthcare NHS Trust, (to be found in Wilkin, 1998a), with the addition of my fictitious names and by kind permission of its author. This contract includes many of the essential and widely accepted components of such documents currently in existence in nursing organisations and is in my view,

---

**ROCHDALE HEALTHCARE N.H.S. TRUST
COMMUNITY MENTAL HEALTH NURSING SERVICE
CLINICAL SUPERVISION CONTRACT** (page 1)

THIS CONTRACT WILL COMPLEMENT THE TRUST POLICY
AND GUIDELINES ON CLINICAL SUPERVISION

SUPERVISEE
NAME: Thomas Knightingale
DESIGNATION: MENTAL HEALTH NURSE (COMMUNITY)

SUPERVISOR
NAME: Helen Florenz
DESIGNATION: CLINICAL SUPERVISOR

VENUE:–
Interview Room, Health Centre.

TIME/FREQUENCY:–
Every two weeks, for one hour. Date and starting time to be negotiated between supervisor and supervisee at the end of each session.

DOCUMENTATION IN CLIENT'S NOTES:–
Supervisee will make an entry in client's notes every time the client is discussed in supervision.

REVIEW OF SUPERVISION:–
Every six months, between supervisor and supervisee. New contract to be signed after the review.

CONFIDENTIALITY:–
As agreed per policy and guidelines on Clinical Supervision

Figure 5.1 *The Rochdale Healthcare NHS Trust clinical supervision contract (page 1)*

an example of good practice in this area and is therefore, at the very least, a useful starting point for the development of clinical supervision contractual documentation. However, nurses intending to draw up such documentation should consider carefully what fundamental information they would wish to be included. I will offer guidance on that matter in the following section, but the ultimate decision needs to be made by those nurses leading the development of clinical supervision in the relevant organisations, with very specific reference to the organisation and its personnel.

CLINICAL SUPERVISION CONTRACT (page 2)
ADDITIONS AND AMENDMENTS

JOINT RESPONSIBILITIES:–

1. To honour the contract

SUPERVISOR'S RESPONSIBILITIES:–

1. To provide supervision as per policy and guidelines.
2. To bring the supervisee's file to each supervision session.
3. To record each client discussed in supervision on a recording sheet after each session.
4. To record caseload management discussion on a recording sheet after the session.
5. To keep the recording sheet safe and confidential outside the session.
6. To end the supervision session.
7. To record each supervision session in the supervision book.

SUPERVISEE'S RESPONSIBILITIES:–

1. To accept supervision as per policy and guidelines
2. To bring case notes and any other material to be discussed to supervision.
3. To accept caseload management a minimum of three times per calendar year.
4. To select suitable clients for presentation at the supervision session.
5. To complete the relevant section on the supervision recording sheet in time for the next supervision session

a) Supervision sessions will only be cancelled due to sickness, or if making the session becomes impossible.
b) If the need for supervision arises outside contracted sessions, a supervisor will accommodate supervisee as soon as possible for an extra session.

NB: The boundaries of confidentiality within supervision are anything that is illegal, breaks the individual's professional code of conduct or infringes the Rochdale Healthcare N.H.S. Trust Disciplinary Policies.

SIGNATURE OF:–

Supervisor . . . . **Date** . . . .

Supervisee . . . . **Date** . . . .

Figure 5.2   *The Rochdale Healthcare NHS Trust clinical supervision contract (page 2)*

The constituents of a clinical supervision contract

The clinical nurse supervisor and her supervisee should discuss some, if not all, of the following issues before the end of the first supervision session and then draw up a contract once its key constituents have been agreed.

THE TIME OF EACH CLINICAL SUPERVISION SESSION

Both clinical supervisor and supervisee should endeavour, as far as possible to arrange a regular and consistent appointment time. If the specific time of each clinical supervision session can be agreed in advance – even for only a few sessions at a time – it will go a long way to allowing the supervisee to feel more supported and secure in his supervision.

THE VENUE FOR EACH CLINICAL SUPERVISION SESSION

Similarly, the place for each session should be agreed in advance and adhered to as far as possible, for as long as possible. Any enforced changes that the supervisor needs to make to the time or venue should be communicated to the supervisee at the earliest opportunity.

THE DURATION OF A CLINICAL SUPERVISION SESSION

The length of each clinical supervision session must be agreed at the first meeting. Once this duration has been agreed both supervisor and supervisee should do what they can to ensure that it is applied to each and every subsequent clinical supervision session. Supervisor and supervisee should try not to let clinical supervision sessions over-run and do what they can to avoid late starting. The clinical supervisor should make herself responsible for 'watching the clock' and ensure that she gently, but firmly, brings the session to a close as soon as possible after the allotted time has elapsed. A useful strategy for good time-keeping in clinical supervision sessions is to keep a clock or watch in sight during the session, perhaps by taking off her wrist-watch and putting it on the desk. The supervisor may wish to announce the amount of time left, as the end of the session approaches. Saying something like, 'We have got ten minutes left, is there anything else you would like say that you haven't already mentioned?' can have the triple effect of warning the supervisee that the session is drawing to a close; guarding against him over-running and helping him to consolidate his thoughts.

A popular time, per individual clinical supervision session for nurses, seems to be that of forty-five minutes. Some nurses trained or training in psychotherapy prefer the so-called psychoanalytic hour, which lasts – somewhat confusingly – for fifty minutes. It is so-called because some therapists with large caseloads, and a requirement to schedule several patients 'back-to-back' in any one day, find it beneficial to leave ten minutes or so between appointments for 'thinking time' and for recording the session.

Building in time to reflect on the session can be a useful method to adopt in clinical supervision practice, no matter what the therapeutic orientation of the supervisor or model of clinical supervision employed. Rather than leaving the room with her supervisee the supervisor can sit quietly for ten minutes or so, pondering the issues raised in the session, and possibly making a list of key words as an aide-mémoire to help her remember the issues at the next session. An extension of this method, which I have adapted from the practice of psychotherapy, is that in the event of the supervisee unexpectedly failing to attend the session, the supervisor can again stay in the room for a short time to reflect on issues raised in the previous session and to ponder on possible reasons for the supervisee's absence. As a guideline, I suggest that clinical supervision sessions should last for *either* one hour *or* forty-five minutes, and that one or the other time is used on a regular basis and that times are not alternated or mixed.

THE FREQUENCY OF THE CLINICAL SUPERVISION SESSIONS

Because the practice is in the comparatively early stages of its development, there are no current 'bench-marks' in terms of clinical supervision session frequency, as it applies to nursing. Nurses practising certain clinical interventions have, in many instances, established a strictly adhered to regime of once-weekly clinical supervision, which may be impracticable and professionally undesirable by nurses from other disciplines.

As a starting point, I would suggest holding clinical supervision sessions every four weeks. Some nurses may prefer a shorter frequency (perhaps meeting every three or even two weeks) and some, either by necessity or through choice, may desire even longer gaps between sessions. Whatever frequency of clinical supervision sessions is agreed, both participants must ensure that they do their best to make certain that this time-scale is maintained.

THE RESPONSIBILITIES OF THE SUPERVISOR

The specific responsibilities undertaken by any clinical nurse supervisor may vary depending on the particular circumstances and people involved and whether supervisor and supervisee agree to share or 'swop' responsibility for particular functions. The majority of functions in this category, however, are ones that cannot be appropriately transferred to the supervisee and will be considered as tasks that most, if not all clinical nurse supervisors can reasonably expect to carry out. A short-list of relevant supervisor responsibilities may include:

Making herself available to the supervisee at the specified time and place and for the full duration of the meeting – without interruption – as previously agreed.

Maintaining the boundary of time by ensuring that the clinical supervision session begins and ends at the stated times.

Ensuring that the supervisee is informed, with as much advance notice as possible, regarding changes to the time, place, postponement and/or cancellation of clinical supervision sessions.

Maintaining the boundary of practice. The supervisor has a responsibility to ensure that her interventions during the specified clinical supervision session time do not fall into any other category than that of clinical supervision. Such inappropriate categories might include management and therapy/counselling.

Maintaining confidentiality regarding the content of the clinical supervision sessions, within the agreed and appropriate limits.

Using her skills of listening, reflection and other intervention skills in the supervisee's best interests and for the promotion of the supervisee's professional development.

Paying and maintaining attention to the content of the supervisee's presentation and challenging any erroneous, irresponsible, negligent, dangerous or in any other way disconcerting content in the presented material or displayed behaviour.

Encouraging the supervisee to seek any specialist help that may be desirable as a consequence of his presentation. This includes advising the supervisee to report any inappropriate and/or unprofessional conduct of himself or others.

Ensuring that she has sufficient professional support and/or clinical supervision of her own in place, in order to prevent being overwhelmed by the role of clinical nurse supervisor.

There is a final boundary I wish to consider, which I call the *boundary of relationship*. I see this particular supervision boundary as one that requires constant vigilance and often a good deal of professional and personal strength, on the part of both the supervisor and her supervisee, to maintain adequately. My rationale for raising this issue is that the friendlier that a working relationship becomes, the more likely it is that the probability of objective professional scrutiny will decrease. My view is that supervisors should not agree to supervise anyone with whom they have (or have had) a close personal relationship. Just how a 'close personal relationship' is defined will, no doubt, be open to conjecture. Some supervisors may choose not to work with any nurse that they are likely to have even limited social contact with. Others will take the definition of 'close personal relationship' to its extreme, and draw the line only at supervising only those nurses with whom they have not had intimate physical contact.

However, Peter Wilkin, a writer and researcher on clinical supervision for nurses, argues that personal relationships between supervisors and supervisees need not necessarily affect the supervisory one. Some of Wilkin's views on the issue of mixing personal and professional relationships in supervision are offered, below.

> I enjoy a social relationship with most of my supervisees – one of them is my best mate! I looked at this issue phenomenologically within a research project (Wilkin 1998a).
> The consensus was that, whilst our social relationships had provided a trusting foundation on which to build our supervisory relationships, our supervisory relationships had actually enriched our 'whole' relationship. My supervisees pointed out that I become 'different' in the supervision session: I leave all my personal agendas outside the room and they feel in no doubt that the 'hour' is theirs to shape and use as they need to, so . . . I don't believe close relationships need automatically rule out adjacent supervisory relationships. I guess it depends on the individuals concerned. (Wilkin, 1999)

I accept that the character, integrity and professionalism of the individuals concerned will be essential factors in determining whether a personal relationship between two people need necessarily negate the prospect of a supervisory relationship between them. Every situation will be different, and needs to be considered separately with, in my view, one stipulation. Namely that only the most experienced of clinical supervisors should ever consider trying to swap their 'friend' hat for their 'supervisor' hat.

THE RESPONSIBILITIES OF THE SUPERVISEE
Clinical supervision is a two-way process and the supervisee also has certain responsibilities to consider, which will help to ensure smooth progress is achieved and maintained. As with those of the supervisor, there are specific responsibilities for supervisees that may need to be agreed on an individual basis, but these are likely to be minimal.

The supervisee should never feel that he is in a position of having to accept whatever form, or standard, of clinical supervision that is offered. He should feel able, and be prepared, to challenge the supervisor's input and direction whenever he feels it necessary. With this in mind a short list of the supervisee's responsibilities, may include:

Ensuring that the content of the supervision session is appropriate to his professional situation.

Making adequate preparation for each clinical supervision session, perhaps by making notes of points he wishes to raise and ensuring that the supervisor is aware of his requirements at the beginning of the session.

Ensuring that the supervisory methods and strategies employed by the supervisor are compatible with the supervisee's level of understanding and professional development.

Ensuring that the supervisor is informed, with as much advance notice as possible, about the supervisee's impending absence from supervision sessions.

Maintaining the 'boundary of time' by ensuring that he arrives ready to start each clinical supervision session on time and planning his presentation in such a way as to avoid over-running the allotted time.

Maintaining the 'boundary of practice' by doing as much as possible to ensure that the development of any external relationship either with the supervisor or others does not interfere with his capacity to benefit from clinical supervision.

Accepting ownership and responsibility for any action he takes as a consequence of the clinical supervision session.

Challenging the supervisor on any comments, advice, suggestions or other input that he regards as inappropriate, inadvisable, unprofessional or in any other way unacceptable.

THE ISSUE OF CONFIDENTIALITY
Another important question that both the clinical nurse supervisor and her supervisee need to consider is:

To what extent will confidentiality be applied and maintained? I believe that all supervisees are entitled to have the issues they raise during clinical supervision protected from being disclosed, casually, to anyone other than the supervisor. If we accept that position, then an important question to consider is, under what circumstances might the supervisor feel compelled to discuss the issues raised by the supervisee, and with whom should she discuss them? I would suggest that clinical nurse supervisors should consider breaking their agreement of confidentiality with supervisees only when they consider that the supervisee has disclosed or demonstrated professional misconduct and/or that they are unfit to continue to practise nursing, for reasons of ill-health.

In addition, the supervisor and supervisee may wish to agree at the outset of the clinical supervision sessions that the supervisor will advise the supervisee to report the misconduct to the relevant authority himself. It should, however, be agreed that the supervisee understands that the supervisor will report the matter if she feels that the supervisee has failed to register his failing at the earliest opportunity.

If these conditions can be understood and agreed at the beginning of the clinical supervision process, it should lead to a more open supervisory relationship in which both participants treat each other as responsible adults.

In the UK, the United Kingdom Central Council For Nursing, Midwifery and Health Visiting (UKCC) publish guidelines for

Complaints About Professional Conduct (UKCC, 1998). The guide-lines contain the following examples of professional misconduct:

1   Physical, sexual or verbal abuse of patients.
2   Stealing from patients.
3   Failing to care for patients properly (for employers and managers registered with the UKCC this can include failing to maintain an acceptable environment of care).
4   Failing to keep proper records.
5   Failing to administer medicines safely.
6   Committing serious criminal offences.
7   Deliberately concealing unsafe practice.

I would advise clinical nurse supervisors to take special note of the final item on this list. It is clear that if supervisors fail to act quickly enough to report instances of professional misconduct on the part of their supervisee, they may well stand accused them-selves.

The most common examples of unfitness to practise for reasons of ill-health, considered by the UKCC (1998) are:

1   Alcohol or drug dependency
2   Untreated mental illness
3   Serious personality disorders

RECORDING THE CLINICAL SUPERVISION SESSIONS
Questions to consider and agreements to make on the matter of the issue of recording the clinical supervision sessions will include:

1   Should a written record be made of the clinical supervision session?
2   Who will make and keep the records?
3   What will be recorded?

Will the clinical supervision session records be made available to anyone other than the clinical nurse supervisor and her super-visee? The recording of information in a professional nursing context is a sensitive and contentious issue. The possible legal and ethical implications of making and keeping records about clinical supervision sessions, therefore, need to be considered very care-fully indeed.

The UKCC Key Statement 6 on clinical supervision states that: 'Evaluation of clinical supervision is needed to assess how it influences care, practice standards and the service. Evaluation systems should be determined locally' (UKCC, 1996). If a reliable evaluation system of the process of clinical supervision is to be established, then some sort of record will need be kept. Professor Bridgit Dimond (1998) has suggested that the employer resourcing the provision of the clinical supervision should have the right to receive: 'the minimum necessary information for effective monitoring to take place'. Dimond further cautions nurses considering setting up clinical supervision systems that: 'if disciplinary proceedings were to be brought against either the supervisor or supervisee then the complete supervision record might have to be made accessible to the employer if it is relevant to an issue arising in the proceedings' (Dimond, 1998: 488). She adds that if the clinical supervision sessions take place during working hours – which is the most desirable option – then the ownership of the records themselves will reside with the employer. Dimond also states that courts are in the position of subpoenaing clinical supervision notes, other than when information is exempt from disclosure on grounds of legal professional privilege.

According to Dimond, patients would also have direct access to clinical supervision records which directly refer to them and if such notes were defined as 'health records' under the Access To Health Records Act (1990), which defines a 'health record as:

> . . . a record which consists of information relating to the physical or mental health of an individual who can be identified from that information and has been made by or on behalf of a health professional in connection with the care of that individual. (Dimond, 1998: 488)

If the supervisor was to record information that named a patient, that person would then have a statutory right of access to the records unless the record-holder – probably the clinical nurse supervisor – could show that viewing them would cause serious mental or physical harm to the individual.

My suggestion for record-keeping, in clinical supervision, is that the supervisor should keep a very brief record of each supervision session, perhaps detailing the following information:

1   The date of the supervision session.
2   The time it began.
3   The time it ended.

4   The names of the people attending the session.
5   A brief note of the issues raised and discussed.
6   The agreed date of the next supervision session.

This record would not contain specific personal information on patients nor any other information that could identify individuals. It has rarely been necessary, in my experience, for supervisees to use more than a person's first name, whether that person was a patient, colleague or other associate. I have also managed to retain enough information about the details of the sessions by using code words or letters of the alphabet, in any records that I have kept.

Some clinical nurse supervisors advise their supervisees to keep a diary of reflective practice to which they can refer during clinical supervision sessions. In addition, supervisees may wish to keep reflective diaries specifically referring to the supervision sessions, as an adjunct to, and a reminder of, the clinical supervision itself. Again, Dimond (1998) warns that such writings may, in certain circumstances, be required to be made available to the courts. It would be unfortunate, in my view however, if concerns of a legal nature prevented supervisors or supervisees from keeping reasonable records of clinical supervision sessions, as many will benefit from a written reminder or aide-mémoire. If supervisors and supervisees take care over what, how and where they record the process of their clinical supervision sessions, it will lead to increased input – and output – and an informed evaluation of the whole process.

WHAT WILL BE DISCUSSED DURING CLINICAL SUPERVISION SESSIONS
Clinical supervision is primarily about one nurse supervising the clinical work of another nurse. If supervisors and supervisees endeavour to keep that in mind, it will be difficult for them to be confused about what should be discussed during the sessions. Clinical supervision – by its very definition – must always have as its focus *a work context* (Hawkins and Shohet, 1989). This means, in essence, that clinical nurse supervisors and their supervisees should talk about anything they want to, so long as it is *always* directly connected to the clinical nursing work of the supervisee.

Butterworth et al. (1997) found that nurses discussed a range of practice-focused issues in clinical supervision sessions including:

Organisational and management issues – such as dealing with changes at work.

Clinical casework – including learning new skills by reflecting on practice.

Professional development – including receiving advice on career development.

Educational support – often concerned with teaching student nurses.

Confidence building – the supervisor may assist the supervisee adjust to new situations and experiences.

Interpersonal problems – such as those related to working in high-pressure environments, team-building problems and organisational development issues.

Personal matters – surrounding the stress and other personal difficulties which arise from or affect the work of supervisees.

WHAT WILL NOT BE DISCUSSED DURING CLINICAL SUPERVISION
SESSIONS
Given the above, it should not be difficult to write a very long list of all the inappropriate issues that supervisees may wish to raise with their supervisors. Put simply, the supervisee should not expect the supervisor to become a 'shoulder to cry on', while he discusses his personal life, his financial problems, the problems he had at school, his last holiday, or the baggage he carries from the break-up of his marriage or the fact that he was abandoned by his parents at birth.

While clinical nurse supervisors should endeavour to be friendly to their supervisees, there is no pragmatic reason why they should become their *friends*. There are important reasons to clarify and maintain the boundaries of the clinical supervision at the very beginning of the process. This includes making sure that both the supervisor and supervisee expect that the focus of the discussions will be on the supervisee and his work and the situations and conditions connected to it. It would be both narrow-sighted and naive to imply that nurses work in a vacuum. No matter how hard we try not to take our private life into work with us, it will inevitably make its way there sooner or later. It would be foolish, therefore, to suggest that nurses should never make any mention of how their work effects them at home or vice versa.

Clinical nurse supervisors must also remember that, whatever their background and qualifications, they are not expected nor entitled to act as a therapist or counsellor for their supervisee. Both supervisors and supervisees need to distinguish between clinical supervision sessions which are primarily focused on work-based issues that might, by necessity cross over into more personal areas of the supervisee's life, and personal and private issues that the supervisee has chosen to raise because there is no one else to talk to about them.

If the supervisor also has a managerial relationship with the supervisee (which I regard as inadvisable, but is often a reality of nursing life) then there should be a firm agreement at the first clinical supervision session that both participants will not discuss any matters that would clearly be appropriate to discuss with the supervisor when she is wearing her manager's hat. In many ways, this can be more difficult than not discussing the supervisee's personal life, because it is often more easily delineated from his professional one. This is not an easy task, which should be avoided, whenever possible, by ensuring that the supervisor is not the supervisee's manager. If such an arrangement is necessary, then both participants should agree to list at the outset of the clinical supervision, which issues will be discussed with the 'manager' and which with the supervisor.

WHAT MODELS AND METHODS WILL THE SUPERVISOR EMPLOY?

Will the supervisor be using a specific model of clinical supervision for nurses? If not, what will be the main methods and theoretical frameworks that the supervisor will employ to aid the supervisee in examination of, and reflection on, his clinical work? No clinical nurse supervisor should attempt to undertake the role without a clear sense of the direction she will be taking, the procedures she will employ and the theoretical reasoning behind them. Although this may seem to some nurses as an unnecessarily meticulous and complex process, I can assure them that unless the clinical nurse supervisor is aware of the general direction and boundaries of her input, the process is likely to become extremely confused and ultimately unworkable.

Clinical supervisors should try to keep – in their heads if nowhere else – a map of where they will go, and where they will *not* go, professionally and theoretically speaking, with any given supervisee. Supervisors must also be able to articulate this mental map to the supervisee, in order that he is able to comment on how his supervisor intends to work with his professional concerns. The supervisor would be wise to consider abandoning the use of certain less usual methods of clinical supervision that the supervisee finds disconcerting, for example, role play or other 'experiential' exercises – rather than risk losing the trust of that supervisee, which could result in him terminating the process.

MECHANISMS FOR NOTIFYING LATENESS, ABSENCE OR ANY OTHER
CHANGES FROM THE PLANNED CLINICAL SUPERVISION SESSION
Many of the points to be considered under this heading are practical issues that require nothing more than the application of common sense and consideration for the other participant. At the first session, the supervisor and supervisee will need to agree on the protocol for notifying each other in the event of certain changes to the agreed supervisory schedule. A short list of such events to consider might include:

• How will the supervisor be told that the supervisee will be arriving late or vice versa?
• How much notice should one participant reasonably expect to be given that the other will not be attending the next scheduled session?
• How will notification of holidays and other expected absences from supervision be given?

The fearful aspects of clinical supervision

Writers on clinical supervision in psychotherapy and social work have highlighted the potential of clinical supervision to become a threatening and anxiety-provoking experience for the supervisee. This sense of being threatened by clinical supervision is likely to occur even if the supervisee is initiating the process himself and appears to understand that it will be an ultimately beneficial experience.

Kadushin (1968) argued that both the supervisee and supervisor can be fearful of, and feel threatened by the prospect and process of clinical supervision in four main ways, which I have adapted to clinical supervision for nurses.

• The supervisee's fear of change
• The supervisee's fear of losing autonomy

- The supervisee's fear of inadequacy
- The supervisor's fear of getting it wrong

I offer an outline of these fears, below, with my thoughts on why they should be regarded as valid concepts in the world of clinical supervision for nurses.

THE SUPERVISEE'S FEAR OF CHANGE
The nursing supervisee is being asked to change even from before the moment he enters the room for his first session. The first – and possibly most disconcerting – change he is faced with, is the prospect of reflecting on his work 'out loud', with his professional knowledge and actions 'laid bare' and open to comment and, possibly, criticism from the supervisor. He may feel that he will no longer be able to disguise or dismiss his frustration with a patient, or mentally brush aside his failure to carry out a nursing procedure exactly to the letter. He may be called upon to do things differently, to give up on the familiar routines that have helped him feel safe about his work – even himself – but which his supervisor may regard as out-moded or inappropriate.

The qualified and experienced nurse may see the concept of change in his working routine as even more threatening than would a student nurse. The experienced nurse will have developed stronger, and therefore more ingrained patterns of thinking and behaving than the novice and it is reasonable to speculate that the more 'expert' in his field of nursing he is, the more threatened he is likely to feel by the idea of engaging in clinical supervision.

THE SUPERVISEE'S FEAR OF LOSING AUTONOMY
My first – abortive – experience of trying to establish clinical supervision for nurses was in the mid 1980s, when I worked as a community mental health nurse. The service I worked within consisted of about eight highly skilled and very experienced nurses. For five days each week – and more if they were on call – they dealt with large caseloads of people often suffering from seriously debilitating mental illnesses, which were often compounded by extremely poor and distressing social and personal circumstances. All of those mental health nurses coped with the most challenging problems with mind-boggling alacrity and reached solutions that frequently left their clients safer and more content and their colleagues – including psychiatrists – in awe of their achievements.

It was common for that team to meet together in the tea-room for half an hour prior to 'going out' for the day, and again at the end of the duty having returned to the office to write their case notes and chat. The 'chat' often consisted of one community mental health nurse describing her visit to a patient. This could be someone with a problem she had not encountered before, or the outline of a particularly stressful, challenging or even humorous event in her day.

What was notable about these 'chats' was that the nurse would offer the information freely, often without invitation and would almost always gladly accept – and frequently invite – comments and suggestions on her experience from any other member of the team. In fact, many of these 'chats' about one nurse's experience grew into vastly enlightening and professionally valuable discussions on the wider issues of coping with a certain type of client, situation or illness and drawing on the varied experiences of the whole team.

In view of these informal discussions and the obvious way in which the team had 'gelled' I suggested that we formally organise the process and instigate regular clinical supervision meetings. The prime intention would be to ensure that each member of the team – and not just those who happened to come back to the office by chance on the evening that an especially useful discussion occurred – benefited from the experience of sharing professional experiences. The team's reaction was little short of hostile. They were certainly against the idea, and I was left with the strong feeling that I had even grossly insulted a number of them. To me, there was no difference in what would happen during a more formal clinical supervision session and what happened in the tea-room – except that the benefits would be felt more regularly and perhaps more evenly distributed among the team. To the team, however, there was a world of difference. There would be less choice about whether to speak about their work and – more importantly – an implied sense of being dependent upon the views of colleagues and more *in need* of their opinion. Those very experienced and skilled nurses, who had no qualms about discussing their work informally over tea, were suddenly faced with the prospect that they might be perceived as less independent and, worst of all, potentially incompetent professionals should they choose to formally discuss their work with others.

The threat that these nurses faced can perhaps be summarised in this way: *If I need to talk, I must need help. If I need help, how can I be considered as capable of working alone. If I am considered incapable of working alone, how can I be regarded as capable of doing my job?*

No matter how illogical that statement may appear as cold type on the page, it is always a very hot issue for those nurses whose independence and autonomy are threatened by the prospect of clinical supervision.

THE SUPERVISEE'S FEAR OF INADEQUACY

No matter how experienced as a nurse the supervisee may be when he arrives for his first clinical supervision session, he is likely to carry into the room with him a concern that something in him is lacking – or could be perceived as being lacking – simply through his very presence in supervision. Supervision, no matter how well-intentioned it may be, has the potential to cause the supervisee to feel 'de-skilled' and unsure of himself professionally. The supervisory situation 'demands an admission of ignorance, however limited, in some areas' (Kadushin, 1968: 24). Kadushin adds that the supervisee also faces the difficulty of feeling that he may not live up to his supervisor's expectations of him, and that he may be disapproved of or even rejected by her.

THE SUPERVISOR'S FEAR OF GETTING IT WRONG

The supervisee is not always alone in feeling threatened by the prospect of failure or inadequacy. The clinical nurse supervisor, particularly if she is inexperienced, will need to have an especially pachydermatous disposition not to feel daunted by the prospect. A concern about doing the right thing by the supervisee – while it should never be allowed to become so intense that it renders the supervisor dysfunctional – could be used to indicate someone with some of the appropriate qualities for conducting clinical supervision. It shows a willingness to consider the possibility of inadequate or inappropriate functioning, which will help the supervisor remain focused on the consequences of her actions, and should indicate that she is prepared to change in the light of the feedback she receives.

I would argue that those who are so insensitive not to ever consider that they might behave in ways that are inappropriate or unhelpful should be steered well clear of clinical supervision responsibility as soon as they express an interest in being considered for the privilege.

A major concern for clinical nurse supervisors who are starting out is knowing what, and how much, to say to the supervisee at any given time in the process. It is this very concern of saying the right thing at the right time that often stops the inexperienced supervisor from saying anything at all, or causes her to hold back from uttering an especially useful view or asking a very pertinent question – with the result that the supervisee loses the opportunity to consider a potentially valuable idea.

Both the supervisor and supervisee will only truly learn from the practical experience of giving and receiving clinical supervision, and the inevitable 'trial and error' nature of the experience. In order that the supervisor becomes more skilled in knowing which of her interventions are useful, which are innocuous and which are potentially disruptive and unhelpful, she needs to make them in the first place. Although this statement is more easily written than done, it may help the inexperienced clinical nurse supervisor to function more effectively if she can accept, and be open to, the prospect of sometimes not getting it quite right.

Think about . . . the worst thing that could happen

Try to bring to mind the worst possible scenario that could happen during clinical supervision, then consider:

1   How strong a possibility is there of your fear becoming a reality?
2   What steps could you take to avoid it happening?
3   If the worst did happen what might be the consequences for yourself?
4   Could you cope with it?
5. If not, why not?

6

Finding a Solution By Knowing How to Look for the Problem!

Key issues in this chapter

- The development of a clinical supervisee
- A framework for supervisory intervention
- The six 'eyes' of clinical supervision

The development of a clinical supervisee

According to Friedman and Kaslow's (1986) 'Six Stage Model of Development of Professional Identity' – originally designed for therapists and adapted to nursing here – a clinical supervisee can be expected to pass through a total of six major stages of personal change and development during the course of a clinical supervision experience. These stages of supervisee development are referred to as:

1 Excitement and anticipatory anxiety
2 Dependency and identification
3 Activity and continued development
4 Exuberance and taking charge
5 Identity and independence
6 Calm and collegiality

Whether the supervisee passes through all of the stages, or only a few of them; how quickly he passes on to the next stage of development or whether he remains stuck at one particular stage will depend on a number of factors, including:

- The length of time spent in supervision.
- The personal make-up of the supervisee.
- The nature of the supervisor–supervisee relationship.
- The skills of the supervisor in identifying the supervisee's current stage of development.
- The skills of the supervisor in facilitating the supervisee's development to the next stage.

Moving through the various stages of development should not be seen as a linear process for the supervisee, but more of a 'circular' one that will be repeated, perhaps at greater levels of understanding. Another important point to stress, is that what I will be describing should be seen as nothing more than a way of trying to paint a rough picture of how the supervisee may think, or feel or behave at certain stages in his supervision. While – like any other model or theory – it can be used as a source of information and guidance, the supervisor should avoid falling into the trap of expecting any given supervisee to behave exactly as described. She should also not assume that there is a problem with either the supervisee or her method of delivering supervision, if the supervisee does not display all of the behaviours in the 'correct' order. I will describe the first three stages here, and the final three will be used to discuss the psychological development and behaviour of the supervisee during the *middle* and *end phases* of clinical supervision, in subsequent chapters.

DEVELOPMENT STAGE 1 – EXCITEMENT AND ANTICIPATORY ANXIETY
The phrase *excitement and anticipatory anxiety* is used to paint a picture of the supervisee at possibly his least experienced, most untrained, most unsupervised and, possibly, his freshest level. Many of the concerns of the supervisee who is starting out will be brought with him into supervision. This first stage of supervisee development is likely, therefore, to be operating even before the first time he enters the supervision room. The inexperienced supervisee wants, most of all, to learn. He is excited by the prospect of gaining new insights into his chosen profession and developing his nursing skills and knowledge. There will be no other time when the supervisee is more motivated and more determined to make the best of the supervision opportunity.

Although the supervisee will be as positively disposed to the process as he is ever likely to be, both he and his supervisor will need to be aware that, perhaps on a deeper, less aware level, the supervisee will also be experiencing a less positive and even potentially dysfunctional response to the process.

Hawkins and Shohet (1989) suggest that inexperienced supervisees can feel anxious and insecure about their role and their own ability to fulfil it. They may also, in my view, lack insight of both their potential strengths and limitations as nurses, and be experiencing some level of anxiety about the process of supervision. Two key areas of anxiety have been referred to by Stoltenberg and Delworth (1987) as *evaluation apprehension* and *objective self-awareness*:

Evaluation apprehension The inexperienced supervisee expects to be judged and criticised. In his worst fantasy – which may operate in such a way that he is not fully aware of it – he knows nothing about nursing at all and expects the supervisor to tell him so immediately. He may even expect, deep down, to be told that he is practising in an unprofessional and/or unsafe manner. In the supervisee's evaluation apprehension fantasy, his supervisor will know all of these things about him instantly and perhaps just from the way he sits in the chair or talks about his work! The supervisee may also be so concerned about making the wrong impression that he becomes unable to do anything at all. An important task for the supervisor, at this stage, is to ensure that she is at least aware of potentially dysfunctional 'evaluation apprehension' in her supervisee.

Objective self-awareness Stoltenberg and Delworth use the term *objective self-awareness* to describe the feelings of anxiety generated in a clinical supervisee when he is aware that the focus of attention is squarely on himself. A supervisee can often feel intimidated simply because he believes he is being scrutinised by the clinical supervisor. Taken to extremes, objective self-awareness can become a negative force as the supervisee becomes conscious of everything he says and does, down to the smallest statement, gesture or mannerism. He may compare himself with other supervisees and make self-effacing or even personally disparaging remarks, in a covert attempt to illicit a favourable comment from his supervisor. The supervisee's concerns about being negatively scrutinised are often increased when he is asked to bring evidence of his clinical work into the supervision session.

An important task for supervisors is to be aware of when they are asking the supervisee to present clinical material in a way that, on the one hand, may be perfectly justifiable and appropriate but, on the other hand, may cause him such anxiety that he is unable to function in a way that is of benefit to himself, or the patient. If inexperienced supervisees are asked to present their supervision material in unusual ways – perhaps through the use of audio or video recordings, written transcripts of the clinical sessions or by use of some experiential work such as role-play – they may become so over-awed and apprehensive about the presentation itself, rather than the material to be presented, that it provides no new insight into his work with the patient. It might be useful for the clinical supervisor to clarify with which particular methods of presentation the supervisee is most familiar. She could then endeavour to use these methods for the supervisee's first few presentations, while at the same time encouraging and preparing him for the use of more elaborate and sophisticated presentation techniques.

DEVELOPMENT STAGE 2 – DEPENDENCY AND IDENTIFICATION
This second stage of development is particularly relevant to newly qualified nurses, who may be beginning supervision at the very outset of their professional careers. The recently qualified nurse-supervisee is likely to be lacking in confidence in his ability to perform tasks as well as his colleagues, and will probably expect his supervisor to be far more experienced, skilled and confident than himself.

Although his nursing education and training may still be fresh in his mind, the new nurse may also consider himself to be far less knowledgeable than his experienced colleagues, working on the assumption that there is much to be learnt that cannot be taught in classrooms. He is therefore also likely to consider his supervisor – especially if she has a number of years' clinical experience behind her – to be far more knowledgeable than himself. There may be a tendency for the new supervisee to see his clinical supervisor, with her experience, knowledge and training as the perfect role-model. He may even begin to think and act like his supervisor, to the extent of mimicking her style of language and behaviour, perhaps copying exact phrases that she uses and the way she sits.

While this may be useful when very new nurses have no other frame of reference on which to base their professional contribution, it can lead to difficulty if the supervisor is not prepared to allow the supervisee to eventually find his own style of thinking and working. No supervisor worth her salt should be taken in by the transient and ultimately meaningless sense of admiration that she will gain from having her supervisee identify with her and proceed to mimic her thoughts and actions. The task of the supervisor, here, is to do what she can to avoid being sucked into the trap of enjoying the adulation too much (although she will be super-human if she does not experience at least a twinge of pride) and concentrate on developing a supervisee with his own distinguishable identity.

New trainees have not had the experience to develop grounded criteria on which to assess their performance and, consequently, can sometimes be dependent on how their supervisor is assessing their work. Supervisees at this stage may expect the supervisor to make the final judgement on whether their work with patients – from the most rudimentary contact, such as greeting a newly admitted person to the ward, to undertaking a comparatively complex nursing procedure – is satisfactory and appropriate.

An important task for the supervisor, here, is to judge when to give the clinical supervisee her direct view on the quality and merits of the work being described, and when to consider asking herself the silent question, *Why am I am being put in this position?* The supervisor may have to consider that the once-useful act of giving her judgement on the supervisee's performance is now causing a problem of not allowing the supervisee to make an independent judgement of his own work. Any clinical supervisor can expect her inexperienced supervisee to want her to offer a view on the quality and standard of his nursing. Indeed, any clinical supervisee who acts as if he knows that everything he does is perfect, or even appropriate, is likely to set alarm bells ringing and needs to be viewed with caution and some concern by his supervisor.

Conversely, the supervisor should refrain from encouraging any supervisee who is displaying a tendency to be unable to function without constant reassurance that his work is satisfactory. All supervisees need to be assisted to a level of functioning that enables them to make a considered and largely accurate assessment of their own practice. The supervisee who asks the supervisor the question: 'I believe I did the best thing possible under the circumstances – would you agree?' can usually be considered to be progressing in his supervisory development faster than the supervisee who simply asks his supervisor: 'Was that OK?'

DEVELOPMENT STAGE 3 – ACTIVITY AND CONTINUED DEVELOPMENT
The time will come, particularly if the supervisor has continued to encourage the principles of independent thinking and behaviour, when the supervisee begins to recognise that he is having a positive influence on his patients. This recognition will bring with it the urge for the supervisee to want to do more for the patients his is working with, and to try out new and increasingly more complex nursing procedures and techniques. He may still feel dependent on his supervisor, to some extent, but he may also be displaying some ambivalence about his supervisor's influence, and will start to display increasingly autonomous behaviour. Hawkins and Shohet state that supervisees at this stage: 'begin to fluctuate between dependence and autonomy and between over-confidence and being over-overwhelmed' (1989: 50).

Much learning takes place during this phase of the supervisee's development. He may begin to see the subtle differences between certain nursing techniques and procedures and to make more informed decisions about the appropriate use of them with particular patients in his care.

A framework for supervisory intervention

It would be unhelpful to suggest that all supervisors should work to a set formula and approach their supervisees in exactly the same way. Similarly, I believe it is wrong to imply that the same approach by a certain supervisor will work with every supervisee that she meets. Perhaps the most useful thing that a supervisor can do is learn to develop a style of her own – through trial and error – and her experience will guide her as to when a certain question or statement will be beneficial for one supervisee but not for another. The problem is that this will take time, and new supervisees are arriving today or tomorrow – not in several years' time when the supervisor has rehearsed and practised her methods in numerous role-playing situations.

In order to breach this supervisory theory–practice gap, a framework for approaching supervision that is easily understandable and practically workable is required. Even newcomers to supervision should be able to implement it from the first session, in order that the process flows smoothly and neither the supervisor nor supervisee are left feeling stuck or embarrassed. Ideally, such a framework needs to be flexible and adaptable enough to withstand the supervisor's professional growth and allow her to continue to use it in different ways with different supervisees who are working not only with different types of patients but also with different levels of clinical experience and knowledge.

In the rest of this chapter, I will begin to outline a framework for clinical nurse supervision that is based on my adaptation and amalgamation of an existing, well-respected model of clinical supervision with an equally valid framework of intervention styles and strategies.

I will offer my thoughts on how a model of clinical supervision originally designed for a range of practitioners including therapists, social workers and counsellors working particularly with people suffering psychological problems, can be adapted to work for nurses. In its original form, the model has the flavour of psychotherapy and incorporates thinking and language best understood by such practitioners. Therefore, I will adapt it to make it more accessible to nurses, who may work with a much wider range of patients, and who may not be familiar with the language of psychoanalysis. I will try to do this, of course, without detracting from the model's original intentions.

No amount of theoretical understanding will ever replace the benefits gained from applying the methods in practice. I suggest that the best way to use any theoretical model is to try it out, in role-play situations at first if necessary, but ultimately where it really counts – with the supervisee.

Two interlocking and complementary systems

Hawkins (1985) and Hawkins and Shohet (1989), described a framework for supervision which considers the process of supervision and the supervisory relationship from six key perspectives. Its authors call the framework by two names: the 'Process Model of Supervision' and the 'Double-Matrix Model of Supervision'. They do this to imply that supervision is concerned not only with what actually happens within the clinical supervision environment itself – the process of clinical supervision – but also that it is composed of two important interlocking systems or matrices, which are called, by Hawkins:

- The therapy matrix
- The supervision matrix

THE THERAPY MATRIX

This relates directly to the nursing relationship and the processes and dynamics occurring between the nurse (supervisee) and the patients. The nurse and his patients are connected in one or more ways depending on the circumstances. Their working relationship may be formalised through an agreed contract, which may be verbal or written, made either with the nurse directly or the organisation generally. This will be demonstrated through the expenditure of time together, on a regular basis performing a shared task – and sometimes by the patient's willingness to comply with the nursing interventions – with the ultimate aim of achieving the stated common goal.

The supervisor assists the supervisee in looking directly at his clinical work with the patients. This usually happens by the supervisee reflecting on the work, either from memory or by using notes. In some cases, supervisees will use audio or even a video-recording of clinical work – depending on the nursing specialism – to aid their reflection.

THE SUPERVISION MATRIX

The second of the two interlocking systems is concerned with the working relationship between the nurse (as the supervisee) and his clinical supervisor and with the processes and dynamics occurring between them. The relationship occurring within the supervision matrix may also be formalised through an agreed contract, verbal or written, probably made, in this case, with the supervisor directly and endorsed by the organisation, and demonstrated through the expenditure of time together, on a regular basis performing a shared task – that of attempting to understand the patient more fully. As in the therapy matrix, the ultimate goal is positive change in the patient. The supervisor assists the supervisee in reflecting on his work with the patients, through the use of the supervision session itself, using the supervisory relationship to generate feelings and ideas that may not be obvious to the supervisee.

Figure 6.1 (adapted from Hawkins and Shohet, 1989) shows how the two main systems of this model combine the professional relationship of the nurse and his patient with that of the nurse (now the supervisee) and his supervisor. The numbers in the diagram indicate how the sub-categories of the model might best 'fit' within the overall model itself. For example, number 1 indicates the 'contents eye' of supervision is situated firmly in the 'nursing matrix' and closely connected to the patient. Most of the

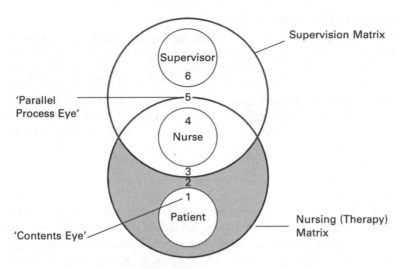

Figure 6.1 *Diagrammatic representation of the Process Model of Clinical Supervision (Hawkins and Shohet, 1989), as adapted to nursing*

issues raised when considering this 'eye' will, therefore, be largely centred around the patient and his direct nursing care. The number 5 (for the 'parallel process eye') suggests a different relationship, in that it is situated between both the 'nursing matrix' and the 'supervision matrix'. It also sits between the supervisee and his supervisor. This indicates that issues raised in relation to this 'eye' should not only link the two matrices together but also that it is concerned with the supervisor/supervisee relationship as much as the patient/nurse relationship.

The six 'eyes' of clinical supervision

An important feature of this model is that each of the two main 'systems' has three sub-categories. The supervisor now has at her disposal two 'general' over-arching ways of thinking about her supervisory tasks and, perhaps more pragmatically, a total of six very distinct approaches to her supervisory activity. She can choose what to do and when to do it, as appropriate. I have chosen to refer to these six sub-categories for potential exploration of specific nursing actions as the six 'eyes' of clinical supervision. I see this particular supervision framework as a way of easily compartmentalising the crucial elements of the supervision process in

Table 6.1   *The six 'eyes' of clinical supervision*

'Eye'	Name of 'eye'	What the supervisor should observe
1	'Content eye'	Content of the nursing interaction
2	'Strategies eye'	Strategies and interventions used by the nurse
3	'Relationship eye'	The nursing relationship
4	'Supervisee's feelings eye'	The nurse's emotional response to the work
5	'Parallel process eye'	How the nursing relationship is reflected in the supervisory relationship
6	'Supervisor's response eye'	The supervisor's own response to the supervision material

terms of what is being considered at any given time. I have outlined the six 'eyes' of clinical supervision in Table 6.1, above, giving the name of the 'eye' and what particular aspect of the supervisee's work the supervisor should be 'looking at' when using it. I will discuss each 'eye' in greater detail in the next section of this chapter.

In my view, the six 'eyes' of clinical supervision do not need to be used in any specific order, and they can work well when used either singly or in conjunction with one and another. I suggest that the supervisor plans her supervisory input in such a way that she begins by using the 'eyes' that will encourage her supervisee to address the issues that are most relevant to him, at the time of the supervisory presentation.

When a supervisee brings a 'new' patient to supervision, the first three 'eyes' can work well in helping to clarify the identity of the patient, his nursing needs and the nature of the nursing relationship, when used in sequence. This can be especially useful when the clinical supervisee is using the supervisory situation to help him think about planning a programme of nursing care.

The six 'eyes' of clinical supervision fit neatly into the three-strand model of nursing supervision functions of Kadushin (1992) and Proctor (1986) outlined in Chapter 3. In Table 6.2, below, I have indicated how each 'eye' might relate to a specific function of supervision. This is something of an arbitrary selection, since what particular meaning or purpose the use of a specific aspect of the model will have, may vary with different supervisees.

Advantages of this model for supervisors of nurses
The 'process model' of clinical supervision (Hawkins and Shohet, 1989) has several advantages for nursing supervisors and their

Table 6.2 *The connection between the eyes of clinical supervision and the main function of supervision*

The 'eyes' of clinical supervision	Main function of supervision		
	Education (Formative)	Support (Restorative)	Management (Normative)
Contents	◉		◉
Strategies	◉		◉
Relationship	◉	◉	◉
Supervisee's feelings	◉	◉	
Parallel process	◉		◉
Supervisor's response	◉	◉	

supervisees. It goes further than some other nursing models in exploring the use of the supervision relationship and the emotional responses of both the supervisor and the supervisee to the work being done and the supervision material being presented in the sessions. Other specific advantages of this model, for nurses, and in my view, are that:

- It is easily understandable and practically workable from the first supervision session.
- It allows the supervision process to flow smoothly and avoids the supervisor and supervisee becoming 'stuck'.
- It is flexible and adaptable enough to withstand the supervisee's professional development.
- It can be used with supervisees with a range of clinical experience and knowledge and working with various types of patients.
- It combines the nursing relationship with the supervision relationship and offers supervisors two over-arching ways of thinking about supervisory tasks.
- It offers supervisors six very distinct approaches, which they can use to be specific about supervisory activity.
- The supervisor can choose what to do and when to do it.
- It can be combined with the stages of supervisee development and adapted to the supervisee's capacity to receive increasingly complex levels of supervision.
- It moves from an 'objective' perspective of the work using the supervisee's presentation of quantifiable and more 'conscious' material (as with the content and strategies eyes), to a more 'subjective' view incorporating the use of the supervisee's emotional responses to the work.

The first 'eye' of clinical supervision: the content of the nursing interaction

This first sub-category – which I call the *content eye* – is concerned with what *happened* in the relationship between the supervisee and the patient. This might be in a very specific sense, such as when discussing a critical incident, or in a less focused sense, as when the supervisee wishes to reflect on his work generally. The 'content eye', in my view, should be unashamedly concerned with the minutia and detail of the nursing relationship, which can be often overlooked or 'passed over' by busy nurses. Clinical supervision is the ideal forum to stop and think about just who this person that we are caring for is, what has happened to them and what they want, in more depth and detail than is usually allowable in the hurly-burly of day-to-day nursing activity.

Hawkins and Shohet state that, although focusing on the details of how things happened between her supervisee and his patients may seem a relatively simple task from the clinical supervisor's perspective, it can appear as a much more difficult and daunting prospect for the supervisee. One particular difficulty for supervisees is that they often try to overcome their anxious sense of *not knowing* what is happening, or how things happened, by rushing in with a premature – and possibly inaccurate – version of events. The supervisor, provoked by her own anxiety, may then compound this initial error, and simultaneously collude with the supervisee, by offering her own solutions and suggestions for what was, in the first place, an erroneous or ill-judged comment. Hawkins and Shohet cite Shainberg (1989) who wrote that true *knowing* comes from:

> being able to observe and describe what is going on in the present in accurate, concrete, and complete detail. This is different from wanting to change or get rid of or compare or assume a fixed meaning about what is happening. (Shainberg 1989: 164)

THE SUPERVISOR'S FUNCTION

Hawkins and Shohet state that in order to fully assist her supervisee to concentrate on the issues raised when using 'the content eye', the clinical supervisor requires: 'the clear focus of a portrait painter or Zen archer'. They add that the supervisor's main task here is: 'to help the supervisees to stay with this difficult task' (Hawkins and Shohet, 1989: 59). In order to do this effectively, the supervisor will need to perform specific and specialised tasks. I offer my adapted list of those tasks below, together with a brief explanation of how it relates to nursing supervision. The first task listed for the supervisor when using her *'content eye'* is, in my view, relevant to all six 'eyes' of clinical supervision and I will examine the purpose of this 'eye' in some detail below and then list the specific details of it for each 'eye' in their relevant sections.

Making links between material from this 'eye' with material from the same 'eye' or other 'eyes' raised in previous supervision sessions   An important task for the supervisor is to ensure that when a supervision session has ended, she and her supervisee do not become 'closed' to the material discussed. There will often be considerable advantage, both to the supervisee and the patients, in referring back to some of this material again in relation to new material raised in subsequent supervision sessions.

I suggest that when using her 'content eye', the supervisor should make statements and ask questions that focus on:

- How the appearances of the patients have changed (or not changed) from one session to another.
- How the physical and psychological condition of the patients have changed (or not changed) from one session to another.
- How a situation involving the patients has changed (or not changed) from one session to another.
- How the requirements, intentions or wishes of the patients have changed (or not changed) from one session to another.
- How interventions from the supervisee – perhaps arising from a discussion of one or more of the other six 'eyes' of supervision – may have changed or in some other way affected the condition, appearance, intentions, requirements and wishes of the patients.

Challenging the supervisee's assumptions   Nurses, because of their experience and training, are capable of making 'expert guesses' about patients and their conditions, needs and wishes. Often these 'guesses', based as they are on other patients in similar situations, are extremely astute. However, when using 'the content eye' of supervision, the supervisor is only concerned with helping her supervisee to present hard fact and correct, indisputable information. Guesses, opinion or assumptions offered by her supervisee, no matter how experienced he may be, are not acceptable. If the supervisee does not have a testable piece of information to hand concerning the patients, he should decide – together with his supervisor – either that it is not relevant to his reflective process or he will seek to clarify the facts. The supervisor's task here, is to challenge the supervisee each time he offers a guess (or assumption) about the patients and to direct him towards thinking about the relevance to the supervisory work of obtaining the facts of the matter.

Helping the supervisee to see the real person in the patient   Patients are individuals in their own right. If the supervisee is to gain a clearer understanding of the person that he is reflecting upon, he needs to avoid using generalisations or 'collective' language. Because of the emphasis of holistic care in current nursing education programmes, fewer nurses these days, I suspect, are likely to be found guilty of referring to the people they care for in such objectionable terms as: 'the hernia in bed four', 'my little old lady with the leg ulcer on Station Road' or 'the suicidal school teacher we admitted last night'. Nevertheless, there is still potential even in a more enlightened nursing environment – and often for good reasons – for supervisees to fall into the trap of seeing the patients they are working with as a 'category' of nursing problem, rather than an individual in their own right. Sometimes it might be 'easier' for nurses to depersonalise the patients than to see them as individuals with families, friends and feelings of their own, simply in order to make the often difficult task of nursing more bearable. The phrase *objectification* was used by Shainberg (1989) to describe what happens when a supervisee decides how the patients should typically behave in order that the clinical work develops along the lines that he expects it to. Supervisees can become angry and disappointed with what has now become simply an 'object' for their clinical skills, if that object does not seem to be responding in a 'text-book' manner. Supervisors must challenge the supervisee's expectations of the patients, particularly when the nursing care fails to produce the expected results, by confronting the supervisee with the reality of the uniqueness of the person that he is reflecting upon. The more the supervisee is capable of regarding the patients as individuals with special characteristics, strengths, needs and wishes the more he will be able to accept diversions from the normal path of progress.

Typical issues   Typical issues that may be raised when the supervisor is assisting her supervisee to concentrate on the content of the nursing interaction can include:

- Who are the patients?
- The physical appearance and physical condition of the patients (including how they dressed, their tone of voice, facial expressions, and gestures).
- The medical/psychological/social condition(s) of the patients.
- What circumstances brought the supervisee and the patients together initially, including reasons for admission to hospital and/or methods of referral to community nursing services as appropriate.
- Where the nursing interaction(s) took place.
- What was said and done by the patients.
- What was said and done by the supervisee.
- The nature of the professional relationship (e.g. the supervisee may be the key worker, the named nurse for the patients).
- The nursing requirements of the patients.
- The stated intentions and wishes of the patients as a consequence of their referral to the nursing services.

Table 6.3 gives possible reasons for use of the 'contents eye' and samples of the types of statements (meta-questions) that the supervisor might make to her supervisee when discussing the supervisee's work in this category.

The second 'eye' of clinical supervision – strategies and interventions used by the nurse

This second sub-category is concerned with exactly what the clinical supervisee *did* in his work with the patients, and I will refer to it as the *'strategies eye'*. It is important that the supervisor and her supervisee understand that it is concerned with *everything* that the supervisee can possibly do when in contact – either directly or indirectly – with patients.

THE SUPERVISOR'S FUNCTION

This 'eye' is closely connected to the educational function of supervision and can be an extremely useful tool for guiding the supervisee towards thinking about and using alternative methods of nursing care.

When using this 'eye' the clinical supervisor is requiring her supervisee to re-examine all of her actions, words and even posture in order to clarify:

Table 6.3 *Samples Box 1 – the first 'eye' of clinical supervision*

The first 'eye' of clinical supervision – content of the nursing interaction

The supervisor's intention		Sample meta-questions
A To establish who are the patients	1	'How much can you tell me about Mr Brown, in terms of his age, marital status, social and personal conditions and his reason for admission/referral?'
B To establish the physical appearance and physical condition of the patients (including how they dressed, their tone of voice, facial expressions, and gestures).	1	'Try to describe Mr Brown physically, perhaps using a famous person as an example.'
	2	'Does Mr Brown appear especially over-weight for his height or perhaps under-nourished and frail?'
	3	'When you meet Mr Brown, does he make good "eye contact" with you, or does he tend to look away, or down at the floor, often?'
	4	'When Mr Brown speaks, is he hard to hear or perhaps too loud at times?'
C To establish the immediate nursing needs of the patients.	1	'Who made the application for admission/ referral for Mr Brown?'
	2	'What do you think that person considers Mr Browns difficulties to be, at present?'
	3	'What would Mr Brown consider his difficulties, if any, to be at present?'
	4	'What do you think are Mr Brown's most urgent nursing requirements, at present?'

- The reasons for its use.
- The consequences of its use.
- Whether he considers that its use was successful or unsuccessful.
- Alternative strategies for use in similar nursing situations or with the same patients.

A useful tool that the supervisor can employ when using the 'strategies eye' is 'brain storming'. I offer, below, the basic rules for brainstorming adapted to the purpose of clinical supervision for nursing:

- The supervisee should say the first thing that comes into his head.
- The supervisor and supervisee should agree to generate as many ideas as possible initially, and then examine them in more detail later.

- The supervisor or supervisee should agree that the ideas raised will not be judged critically but rather, evaluated on their merits as suitable nursing strategies.
- The supervisor and supervisee should agree that any ideas raised in the first instance may be used as springboards for other, more advanced ideas.
- The supervisor and supervisee should agree that any idea no matter how outrageous it may appear at first can be considered as suitable for examination and/or modification as appropriate.

Typical issues A common problem for clinical supervisees is one that Hawkins and Shohet call 'dualistic thinking', by which they mean that supervisees often find it difficult to move out of an 'either-or' way of thinking about their clinical work. In nursing supervision, dualistic thinking can be observed when the clinical supervisee expresses his view about the progress about his work with the patients in a way that suggests that there is only one alternative action for example:

- 'Either he complies with treatment or he will be discharged.'
- 'Either I pass the course or I will be considered unsuitable as a community nurse.'
- 'She talks so much that all I can do is either interrupt her and seem rude, or wait until she has finished and worry about missing or forgetting something that she has said.'
- 'Either I am always early in arriving for my shift, or I will be considered unreliable.'
- 'I feel as if I have to agree with everything that she says or I will be seen as argumentative and unhelpful.'

Hawkins and Shohet refer to the sort of thinking above as 'restrictive assumptions' and state that the function of the supervisor is to avoid the trap of helping the supervisee evaluate between these two choices, but rather to point out how they have reduced numerous possibilities to only two. They suggest that when the supervisee realises that he is being negatively influenced by his restrictive assumption, the supervisor will be in a position to help him generate new strategies and interventions for use with the patients.

Table 6.4 gives possible reasons for use of the 'stategies eye' and samples of the types of statements (meta-questions) that the

Table 6.4   *Samples Box 2 – the second 'eye' of clinical supervision*

The second 'eye' of clinical supervision – strategies and interventions used by the nurse

The supervisor's intention	Sample meta-questions
A To establish the conditions under which the nursing interaction(s) took place.	1 'It would be helpful if you could describe exactly where you were when you met Mr Brown.' 2 'I was wondering if you were both seated, both standing or one sitting and one standing?' 3 'Do you suppose the conditions of your meeting had any bearing on what happened or the consequences?'
B To establish what was said and done by both the supervisee and the patients.	1 'It would be helpful if you could tell me what Mr Brown said to you and how you responded, trying to remember as much of the original language as possible.'
C To encourage the supervisee to consider the consequences, for the patients, of the use of a particular nursing strategy.	1 'I was wondering what Mr Brown thought of what you did.' 2 'If Mr Brown had a choice, do you think he would want you to do something else next time?' 3 'On reflection, do you think you did the most appropriate thing, under the circumstances?'
D To encourage the supervisee to consider possible alternative strategies for use in similar nursing situations or with the same patients.	1 'You said that you suggested to Mr Brown that he spoke to his wife about the matter. Could there be anything else that you might want to suggest to him that might be even more effective?' 2 'Would you want to do anything differently, in a similar situation with Mr Brown or another patient?' 3 'I was wondering if you would do that again with Mr Brown or someone else, if you were faced with a similar situation, or whether you would try something else?'
E To encourage the supervisee to consider his use of 'dualistic thinking' and the problems that he might be facing because of it.	1 'It seems to me that you believe that you only have an "either-or" choice of things you can do, in this situation, with Mr Brown. Is that how it really feels for you?' 2 'It would seem, from the way you describe it, that you can only do one of two things, in this situation, and that there is no possible third way of looking at the problem. Does it seem like that to you, too?' 3 'The choice you are faced with seems to be between two extremes. Is it possible that there may be some 'middle-ground' into which you can move with Mr Brown, at present?'

supervisor might make to her supervisee when discussing the supervisee's work in this category.

The third 'eye' of clinical supervision – the nursing relationship

When using what I will refer to as 'the relationship eye' of supervision, the supervisor is concerned with what happened when the nurse and his patient came together in a professional relationship. When using her 'relationship eye' the supervisor is looking beyond the detail and facts and figures she is concerned with when using either her 'content' or 'strategies' eyes. She is particularly interested in those things that cannot be so easily quantified but which add colour and definition to the outline sketch the supervisee has already drawn. Unusually, perhaps, for some nurses the 'relationship eye' is used to look at the special nature and characteristics of the nursing relationship which are not necessarily obvious when looking with either the 'contents' or the 'strategies' eyes. The 'relationship eye' uses a medium of 'poetic' and metaphoric language that may be unfamiliar, and potentially daunting, to nurses more used to hard facts. It is not an easy task for nurses primarily involved with the physical care of people to begin to think about what they do or what is happening between themselves and those people in anything other than the efficient language of nursing. Indeed, the notion that there might be any form of 'relationship' other than the obvious nursing one between themselves and their patients will often be a hard pill to swallow for some nurses.

Nurses trained to understand and use the concepts of psychoanalytic or psychodynamic therapy, are more used to viewing the nursing relationship in such a way and it often becomes an integral part of their clinical activity. Such nurses will often discuss their professional relationships using the technical terms of *transference* and (the even more difficult to spell) *countertransference*. Transference is a word originally devised by Sigmund Freud (1915) which can be used to describe the process by which the patients can pass on to the nurse feelings, attitudes and attributes which are not truly appropriate to that nurse but which, more properly, belong to a significant attachment figure in the patient's past. The feelings, attitudes and attributes transferred can be either positive or negative and usually are actually meant for a parent or other close relation, such as a brother or sister. Although these transferred feelings are likely to be transient in nature, they can also appear to be very powerful and intense from the position of both the patient and the nurse on to whom they are being transferred.

THE SUPERVISOR'S FUNCTION

An important task for the supervisor when using her 'relationship eye' is to assist her supervisee to colour in the picture of the patient that he has already sketched from the use of the first two 'eyes'. She can do this with a range of questions, similar to the ones suggested below.

- What is the history of the nursing relationship?
- How did you first meet the patient?
- How did you become directly involved with the nursing care of this person?
- What did you first notice about this person?
- How do they see you? Perhaps in terms of a family figure (e.g. are you a kind of mother/father figure, big sister/brother, little sister/brother, aunt or uncle).
- How do they see you in a metaphorical sense? (For example, are you a kind of: 'guardian angel/angel of mercy', 'prison warder', 'the grim reaper' or 'torturer'?)
- How do they feel about you – are they mainly positive, negative or indifferent?

Some writers on clinical supervision use the phrase 'helicopter view' to suggest a way that the supervisee might view the relationship between himself and the patients. As can be imagined, this entails some distancing and objectivity, often not an easy task given the intensity of the work and the strong feelings generated by it at times. The supervisor needs to find techniques that she can employ with her supervisee which will allow him to see both the patients and himself as if he were sitting alongside her in a helicopter and observing himself and his work from a distance. Hawkins and Shohet (1989) recommend three techniques that encourage distancing and detachment in the clinical supervisee:

- Encouraging the supervisee to find an image or metaphor to represent the relationship.
- Encouraging the supervisee to imagine the kind of relationship he would have with the patients if they met in other circumstances or if they were both cast away on a desert island.

- Encouraging the supervisee to think of himself as a fly on the wall at the last meeting with the patients.

Typical issues It is not uncommon for supervisees to be confused about why their work with patients has become difficult or why the person they are caring for seems to be responding in an altogether inappropriately negative or positive way towards them. If a patient expects all nurses to disregard his wants and needs and to be more interested in others than himself it is possible that she will then treat the nurse in a disparaging way and be critical of any attempts on behalf of the nurse to attend to his own needs. Because the nurse is only human, it is not out of the question that he will eventually stop trying to please the patient which will lead to 'confirmation' that she was right about him all along.

Through the use of the 'relationship eye' it is possible for the supervisor to assist the supervisee in gaining some insight into such complex issues, but only if both parties are prepared to approach the nurse/patient relationship from a perspective that may be unfamiliar to either or both of them.

In order to use this 'eye' successfully the supervisor should learn techniques which will allow her and her supervisee to brainstorm ideas around the nursing relationship. Such brainstorming might include comments and suggestions from the supervisor along the lines of:

- Think about how this person will discuss you to his friends and relatives.
- Would this person speak to you if you met at a party? What would they say?
- Is it possible you remind this person of anyone in their family?
- Does this person have a 'general' opinion of nurses? What is it? Does it apply to you?
- If this person knew you socially do you think he would want to make you a friend or would he say that you are someone that he would avoid, and why?

Table 6.5 gives possible reasons for use of the 'nursing relation-ship eye' and samples of the types of statements (meta-questions) that the supervisor might make to her supervisee when discussing the supervisee's work in this category.

Table 6.5   *Samples Box 3 – the third 'eye' of clinical supervision*

The third 'eye' of clinical supervision – the nursing relationship

The supervisor's intention		Sample meta-questions
A To encourage the supervisee to consider the value of the nursing relationship from the perspective of the patients.	1	'Under what circumstances did you first meet Mr Brown?'
	2	'Is it likely that the circumstances of your first meeting with Mr Brown could have "set the scene" for the way you relate to each other?'
B To help the supervisee to consider the existence and possible meaning of any underlying significance to the nursing relationship for the patients.	1	'Is there a history to this particular nursing relationship?'
	2	'How did you become directly involved with the nursing care of Mr Brown?'
	3	'What did you first notice about Mr Brown?'
C To encourage the supervisee to consider how the patients might value the professional relationship with the nurse by likening it to a 'stereotypical' family or personal relationship.	1	'Is it possible that Mr Brown sees you as a kind of big brother, or perhaps some other kind of family member?'
	2	'Think about how Mr Brown will discuss you to his friends and relatives.'
	3	'I wonder what Mr Brown would say if he met you at a party?'
D To encourage the supervisee to consider how the patients might experience the nursing relationship in a metaphorical or 'broad' sense.	1	'Do you think that Mr Brown would have a "general" opinion of nurses? What is it? Does it apply to you?'
	2	'Is it possible that Mr Brown sees nurses, generally, in a certain way – as "angels of mercy" or less positively as "prison warders" or in some other stereotypical way, perhaps?'
	3	'If Mr Brown knew you socially do you think he would want to make you a friend or are you someone that he would avoid, and if so, why?'

The fourth 'eye' of clinical supervision – the nurse's response to the work

This fourth method of viewing the work of the nurse – what I will call the 'supervisee's feelings eye' – is one that the supervisor can use to help her supervisee to understand, more fully, how he feels about the patients and the work that he is doing with them. This 'eye' is closely connected to the 'supportive' (or 'restorative') aspect of supervision and can therefore perform the dual function of offering the supervisee insight into his work and simultaneous support and understanding for the strain that it will inevitably put upon him. The term countertransference, was also originally coined by Sigmund Freud (1910), and can be used to describe the feelings and attitudes that are generated *in the nurse*, about the patients, and the work he is doing with them. In essence, the nurse will respond either knowingly or unknowingly, to what the patient thinks of him or does to him.

THE SUPERVISOR'S FUNCTION

When using this 'eye' to observe the clinical work of her supervisee the supervisor should try to assist her supervisee in examining the feelings that he has for the patients and the work he is doing with them from four main perspectives:

1   Any feelings that the supervisee may have about the patients which can either be associated to the supervisee himself, or his own past life or current situation and which can be identified with the life or situation of the patients.

Typical statements or questions that the supervisor can use to assist her supervisee in uncovering such feelings in himself might include:

'Do you have anything in common with Mr Brown?'

'Does Mr Brown do anything that reminds you of yourself?'

'Does Mr Brown do anything that particularly annoys or irritates you?'

'Could there be a link with what is happening or has happened to Mr Brown with something from your own life, either recently or in the past?'

'Is it possible that Mr Brown's experience, as you understand it, is reminding you of something that you may have forgotten about yourself?'

2   Any feelings that the supervisee may have about the patient that could be a direct result of the feelings that the patient may be expressing towards the supervisee.

Typical statements or questions that the supervisor can use to assist her supervisee in uncovering such feelings in himself might include:

'You say that you are feeling protective towards Mr Brown and defending his behaviour to the rest of the nursing team. Is it possible that by doing so, you are responding to his need to have you as a big brother/sister?'

You say that you sometimes feel emotionally exhausted after nursing Mr Brown. Is it possible that you are responding to his difficulty in co-operating with you, in his nursing care?

You have described feeling very warm and positive towards Mr Brown. Could it be that you are responding to his need to be loved and cared for, perhaps as a parent or a partner would care for him?

3   Any feelings that the supervisee may have about the patient that might be used by the supervisee to protect himself against the feelings, or the situation, of the patient.

Typical statements or questions that the supervisor can use to assist her supervisee in uncovering such feelings in himself might include:

'You tell me that Mr Brown is someone that you find hard to be with for more than a few minutes. Is it possible that this is connected with the fact that he is suffering a great deal and although you feel for him, it could be your way of trying to remain emotionally uninvolved?'

'You tell me that you find Mr Brown objectionable. Is it possible that this feeling is connected to the fact that he may be emotionally attached to you, in some way that neither of you fully understand, and this feeling that he is objectionable is your way of avoiding responding too positively towards him in return, in order to maintain a professional distance?'

'You tell me that Mr Brown makes you feel angry. What would be the opposite feeling to *angry* for you and why is it that you can't feel that about Mr Brown at the moment?'

4   Any feelings that the supervisee may have that might be an indicator of how the patients are actually feeling themselves, either physically or emotionally.

A typical statement that the supervisor can use to assist her supervisee in uncovering such feelings in himself might be:

'You tell me that although Mr Brown seems relaxed and in good spirits when you meet, you often feel miserable or sad either during your time with him or immediately afterwards, with no obvious reason. Is it possible that Mr Brown might also be feeling miserable or sad, deep down inside himself, and that you are somehow picking this up about him, even though he might not realise it himself?'

Typical issues   Sometimes, nurses will want to brush off and avoid any strong emotions at all that may arise during the course of their work. Sometimes this can be because the idea that they are feeling anything other than 'appropriate concern' for the people in their care can leave them feeling unprofessional or 'wrong' in some way. This sense of feeling 'wrong' can be heightened if the feelings that nurses experience in relation to patients are especially warm and positive or especially cold and negative.

Table 6.6 gives possible reasons for use of the 'nurse's response eye' and samples of the types of statements (meta-questions) that the supervisor might make to her supervisee when discussing the supervisee's work in this category.

Think about . . . transference and countertransference in the nursing relationship

Psychoanalytic theory holds that there may be things happening in the clinical situation – between the patient and the nurse – that one (or both) of them may not be fully aware of . . .

1 Are there some patients that you would prefer to nurse than others?
2 Are there some patients that leave you feeling tired and drained just from speaking to them for more than a few minutes?
3 What do the patients in (1) have that those in (2) do not have (and vice versa).
4 Have you ever felt . . . angry, sad, happy, irritated, frustrated for absolutely no obvious reason when talking to a patient?
5 How many patients have made you feel that they want you to be their mother/father/sister/friend without ever coming right out and saying it?

The fifth 'eye' of clinical supervision – how the supervisory relationship mirrors the nursing relationship

An interesting phenomenon of supervision, originally suggested by the psychoanalyst Harold Searles (1955) – which he originally called the 'paralleling phenomenon' – is that the personal responses of the patients to the nurse, may not be confined to the nursing relationship and may be seen to be 'mirrored' (or 'paralleled') in the nurse's relationship with his supervisor. This pattern of mirroring is not necessarily one that the nurse is aware of, as it is often an 'unconscious process' (Freud, 1915) and it may happen when the supervisee is particularly 'stuck' in his work with the patients, or unable to express a feeling or idea by any other means than by demonstrating it through his unconscious actions.

Table 6.6   *Samples Box 4 – the fourth 'eye' of clinical supervision*

The fourth 'eye' of clinical supervision – the nurse's response to the work

The supervisor's intention	Sample meta-questions
A To encourage the supervisee to become aware of any feelings that he may have about the patients which can either be associated to the supervisee's own past life or current situation and which can be identified with the life or current situation of the patient.	1 'Is it possible that you might have anything in common with Mr Brown?' 2 'I was wondering if Mr Brown does anything in particular that reminds you of yourself?' 3 'It's just a guess, but perhaps you find Mr Brown particularly annoying at times, or maybe there is a better word to describe what he does to you?' 4 'Could there be a link with what is happening or has happened to Mr Brown with something from your own life, either recently or in the past?' 5 'Is it possible that Mr Brown's experience, as you understand it, is reminding you of something that you may have "forgotten" about yourself?'
B To encourage the supervisee to become aware of any feelings that he may have about the patient that could be a direct result of the feelings that the patient may be expressing towards the supervisee.	1 'You say that you are feeling protective towards Mr Brown and defending his behaviour to the rest of the nursing team. Is it possible that by doing so, you are responding to his need to have you as a big brother/sister?' 2 'You tell me that that you sometimes feel emotionally exhausted after nursing Mr Brown. Is it possible that you are responding to his difficulty in co-operating with you, in his nursing care?' 3 'You have described feeling very warm and positive towards Mr Brown. Could it be that you are responding to his need to be loved and cared for, perhaps as a parent or a partner would care for him?'
C To encourage the supervisee to become aware of any feelings that he may have about the patient that might be used by the supervisee to protect himself against the feelings, or the situation, of the patient.	1 'You tell me that Mr Brown is someone that you find hard to be with for more than a few minutes. Is it possible that this is connected with the fact that he is suffering a great deal and although you feel for him, it could be your way of trying to remain emotionally uninvolved?' 2 'You tell me that you find Mr Brown objectionable. Is it possible that this feeling is connected to the fact that he may be emotionally attached to you, in some way that neither of you fully understand, and this feeling that he is objectionable is your way of avoiding responding too positively towards him in return, in order to maintain a professional distance?'

Table 6.6   *continued*

The fourth 'eye' of clinical supervision – the nurse's response to the work

The supervisor's intention	Sample meta-questions
	'You tell me that Mr Brown makes you feel angry. What would be the opposite feeling to *angry* for you and why is it that you can't feel that about Mr Brown at the moment?'
D To encourage the supervisee to become aware of any feelings that he may have that might be an indicator of how the patients are actually feeling themselves, either physically or emotionally.	1 'You tell me that although Mr Brown seems relaxed and in good spirits when you meet, you often feel miserable or sad either during your time with him or immediately afterwards, with no obvious reason. Is it possible that Mr Brown might also be feeling miserable or sad, deep down inside himself, and that you are somehow picking this up about him, even though he might not realise it himself?'

What may happen, in essence, is that the supervisee 'carries', in his head, a situation that is occurring between himself and the patient that he is working with, into the supervision session. Because the supervisee has not yet fully understood the situation, or even that *it is happening at all*, it can often appear as if the supervisee is bringing a situation to supervision that actually has its roots in the relationship between the supervisee and his supervisor.

The phenomenon originally described by Searles and now almost universally referred to as 'the parallel process', has become an important aspect of supervision particularly for those working in psychodynamic psychotherapy. Although it has been researched a number of times in recent years the most extensive study on the parallel process was undertaken by Doehrman (1976), who examined its effects in the supervision of psychotherapists. An important finding of Doehrman's study was that the parallel process was present in every three-way professional relationship (supervisor-supervisee-patient) that she examined (Mayman, in Doehrman, 1976).

I will refer to the fifth 'eye' of supervision for nurses as the 'parallel process eye'. With it, the supervisor is able to view the relationship between her supervisee and the patients from directly within the supervision relationship itself. Hawkins and Shohet (1989) state that this function serves two purposes for the

supervisee: one is that it is a form of discharge – 'I will do to you
what he has done to me and you see how you like it' – and the
second is an attempt to solve the problem through re-enacting it
within the supervision relationship.

Boyd (1978: 42), has described the parallel process as: 'one of the
most interesting dynamic patterns in . . . supervision'. He states that
the pattern consists of the supervisee replaying, within the supervisory setting, significant dynamics of the helping relationship.
Common instances of this pattern of behaviour in supervision,
might include:

- The patient expressing dependence on the nurse and the
  nurse expressing dependence on his supervisor.
- The patient becoming angry with the nurse and the nurse
  becoming angry with his supervisor.
- The patient dominating the nurse and the nurse then attempting to dominate his supervisor.

Searles (1955) and later Hora (1957) both stressed that the parallel
process was an unconscious identification with the patient by the
supervisee. Searles felt that the unconscious identification assisted
the supervisee with the reflection process and stated: 'It is as if the
(supervisee) were unconsciously trying, in this fashion, to tell the
supervisor what the (nursing) problem is' (Searles, 1955: 109).
Hora suggested that the supervisee sometimes automatically and
involuntarily adopts the patient's tone of voice and behaviour to
help convey to the supervisor emotions that are experienced by
him during the nursing relationship. For the supervisor, it can be
more like sitting with the patient than with the nurse. According
to Searles, the feelings that the supervisee has about the patients,
and those that he reflects in the supervision session, are outside
his awareness until they are described by the supervisor. At that
point they can become something that the supervisee can use to
the benefit of the patients, rather than the block to his work with
both the patients and also his supervisor that they may have been
previously.

THE SUPERVISOR'S FUNCTION
It is not, of course, out of the question that if the supervisee raises
an issue which seems to be between himself and his supervisor
that it is exactly that, and that there is no hidden meaning or
agenda attached to it. At other times, though, things that happen

between the supervisee and his supervisor may be more complex than they first appear. They may, indeed, be 'coded' examples of either how the supervisee feels about a situation that has happened between himself and his patient and/or a difficulty with the nursing relationship that he has not yet fully explored and understood.

An important function for the supervisor, when using her 'parallel process eye' is, therefore, to point out to the supervisee that he may be bringing issues to supervision that appear, at first sight, to be about – or directly related to – himself and his supervisor, but which, on further investigation can be shown to be 'mirror images' of the nursing relationship, which have yet to fully understood.

Loganbill et al. (1982) stress that supervisors should become aware of the importance of understanding the function and existence of the parallel process because it is in this way that some of the most potent supervisory interventions can be made. McNeill and Worthen agree that the parallel process in supervision, in its various manifestations, can be: 'the focus for some of the most potent and impactful interventions within the supervisory relationship' (1989: 333). They suggest that supervisors pay close attention to the process in order to facilitate effective supervision. Boyd, however, believes that reasons for the occurrence of the parallel process are open to debate and states that it may, in itself:

> . . . be no more than happenstance, since the main dynamic dimensions of human relationships are few and universal and possibilities exist that a certain percentage of instances would illustrate similar dimensions that could be interpreted as [the parallel process]. (Boyd, 1978: 42)

Proper use of the 'parallel process eye' requires the supervisor to display a great deal of self-awareness, professional honesty and a capacity to admit mistakes. Use of this 'eye' can easily become an excuse for the supervisor to divert attention – and the fact that she may be in some way responsible to the supervisee – away from herself and use it to confuse the supervisee with irrelevant jargon and, what some nurses refer to as, 'psycho-babble'. If the outcome is to be effective and to the benefit of the patients, the supervisor must be prepared to implement the following actions each time that she uses her 'parallel process eye' to observe the work of her supervisee:

- The supervisor must be prepared to constantly monitor and examine her actions in the supervision sessions to the benefit of her supervisee and the patients.
- The supervisor must be prepared, having monitored and reflected upon her actions within the supervision sessions, to accept that material presented by the supervisee which appears to relate directly to herself and her actions in the supervision sessions may actually do so, and then to act accordingly to redress the situation.
- The supervisor must also be prepared, having monitored and reflected upon her actions within the supervision sessions, to accept that material presented by the supervisee which appears to relate directly to herself and/or her relationship with her supervisee may, in fact, be a mirroring of the relationship between the supervisee and the patients, but of which the supervisee is currently unaware.

I believe that use of the 'parallel process eye' by the clinical supervisor should (and often does) contain the following characteristics:

- It should be used to observe the behaviour of the supervisee and/or his interaction with his supervisor in order to 'see' something about the patients and their relationship with the supervisee, which may not be obvious to either the supervisor or her supervisee otherwise.
- It should create a shift away from what the supervisee might otherwise have said or done about the patients.
- The use of the 'parallel process eye' should create a new way of thinking about the nursing problem that is ultimately beneficial to both the supervisee and the patients.

Typical issues I first became aware of the possibility of the phenomenon of the parallel process in supervision some years ago, when supervising two community mental health nurses together in a small group, (Power, 1994a). Clare, an experienced nurse, had been describing her work with Jane (a woman in her late twenties who had experienced a series of difficult relationship problems and was now suffering from clinical depression) to the other supervisee, David, and myself.

Clare had seemed exasperated, stating that although Jane had seemed to appreciate that the best way to a solution was through reflection on her difficulties – and ultimately finding her own answers – she was constantly looking to Clare for direct solutions to her problems, without ever trying to work on them herself. Clare had offered several carefully thought-out strategies (assisted by the use of the second 'eye' in supervision) to try and help Jane to find her own answers but had met with little success. Despite being thwarted by Clare's rebuttals and obvious unwillingness to solve her problems, Jane had expressed no anger directly at Clare, but, instead, failed to attend her last scheduled appointment. We discussed Jane's difficulty in expressing anger directly to those that she also looks to for help and caring in her life – both past and present. It seemed possible that Jane was feeling let down by Clare, and that her absence that week could be understood as an expression of her anger, which she would never have been able to show directly, for fear of the dire consequences (i.e. being rejected by Clare and possibly having her care terminated). No sooner had we discussed these issues, with some obvious agreement between the three of us, than Clare expressed some empathy with Jane, saying that she felt sad that Jane had obviously not got the answers that she needed, and could understand how she may be feeling let down. As she said this, Clare looked me straight in the eyes, with a stare which I feel sure, with the benefit of hindsight, was meant to express her intense dissatisfaction with me – at the very least! David, whom I assumed had also noticed Clare's gaze, commented that she might, like Jane, *also* be feeling let down – but in Clare's case by supervision – because she had not got enough from it to enable her to help Jane. Clare replied, laughing, 'You may be right.' I told Clare that she might be feeling *particularly* angry with me, given that I was her clinical supervisor and I was the one in a position to *help* her just as she was in a position to *help* Jane. I suggested that perhaps I had not given her enough of the 'answers' to assist her in helping Jane, during the course of the supervision.

Clare's expression and posture changed again, as she dramatically folded her arms and glowered intently at me before saying, in an icy-cold voice: 'Yes, I am angry. You are my clinical supervisor, but you don't ever tell me *what* to do, even though you have the most experience in this group. I have been looking to you for some answers to Jane's problems for some time now and I still haven't got them!'

I paused for a short time, after Clare stopped speaking, to allow the three of us time to consider the possible *meaning* of what she had just said in the silence before replying: 'It's just a guess but I wonder if Jane might be feeling in a similar way towards you, as you are feeling towards me at the moment? As an experienced Mental Health nurse, you are aware of the value of allowing people to find their own answers to problems, and you have been careful to work in that way with Jane but perhaps it hasn't stopped Jane from being angry because she feels you could have done more for her? During our supervision I have worked in a similar way with you, allowing you to reflect on your work and find your own answers as far as possible. But, even though you seem to understand the reasons for why I work in this way and appreciate the value of my methods, it still hasn't prevented you from being angry with me. In some ways, I think you might be telling us just how Jane is feeling about you. The main difference is that you have expressed the feelings directly, but she has expressed them in an indirect, and possibly less satisfactory way, because she is afraid of your response.'

This was the first time that I had personally experienced the powerful effects of what I later understood as 'parallel process'. It is perfectly possible, of course, that there was no connection between Clare and Jane's nursing relationship and our supervision meeting and that I had fabricated the links between the two apparently disparate situations. However, it made sense to Clare and she was able to use the experience to help Jane with her difficulties during the rest of the time that she was her key nurse.

Table 6.7 gives possible reasons for use of the 'parallel process eye' and samples of the types of statements (meta-questions) that the supervisor might make to her supervisee when discussing the supervisee's work in this category.

The sixth 'eye' of clinical supervision – the supervisor's response to the supervision

The sixth 'eye' of supervision is directly concerned with how the supervisor herself responds to the material that the supervisee brings to the sessions. When using what I will refer to as her 'response eye' the supervisor is in a position to offer insights on the work of her supervisee that may not have otherwise been possible or considered by any other means. The particular response that the supervisor has when listening to her supervisee may take many forms including:

- Hunches, intuitions, gut feelings and guesses about the supervisee's work.

Table 6.7   *Samples Box 5 – the fifth 'eye' of clinical supervision*

The fifth 'eye' of clinical supervision – how the supervisory relationship mirrors the nursing relationship

The supervisor's intention	Sample meta-questions
A To suggest to the supervisee that he may be offering a 'coded' example of a difficulty within the nursing relationship that he has not yet fully explored and understood.	1 'You seem to have been asking me to offer you very specific direction and guidance with your nursing care of Mr Brown, which is unusual for you. I wonder if that can tell us something about how Mr Brown expects you to act in your nursing care of him?'
	2 'I noticed that you missed our last supervision appointment, and that in the session you had been telling me that Mr Brown was having problems complying with his nursing care plan. It's just an idea, but perhaps you were giving me a "taste" of how frustrating it feels for you to be on the receiving end of such behaviour.'
	3 'I have found it difficult to "get a word in edge-ways" with you lately. It is almost as if I do say something, you will find it too controlling or restricting, perhaps? I wonder if you have felt like that about your work with Mr Brown lately, too?'

- Recalled memories and/or thoughts relating either to her work with this supervisee, other supervisees or her own clinical work.
- A sudden and often inexplicable emotional reaction, which can include feelings of: anger, apathy, tiredness, boredom, sexual arousal, excitement, confusion, disappointment, elation, amusement, sadness and anxiety.

Some supervisors might find the notion of expressing their feelings in this way as, at best, unusual or, at worst, unprofessional. However, the supervisor's 'response eye', when used carefully, can offer important insights on the feelings of either her supervisee and, in particular, the patients which have yet to be fully recognised.

THE SUPERVISOR'S FUNCTION

When using her 'response eye', the supervisor is making use, at least to some extent, of the psychodynamic concept of counter-transference (Freud, 1910) in a very similar way to which she will encourage her supervisee to use it when examining his work with the 'supervisee's feelings eye'. The difference, here, is that it is the supervisor who is encouraged to think about the feelings generated by the work and to use these feelings, or just as importantly, to decide not to use these feelings to offer insight on the work of her supervisee.

In order for the 'response eye' to operate the supervisor needs to regularly monitor her feelings and responses to the clinical supervisee, with as much professional honesty and self-awareness as used for the fifth 'eye'. The more self-aware the supervisor is, the more likely it is that she will be able to recognise feelings of anger, apathy, tiredness, boredom, sexual arousal, excitement, confusion, disappointment, elation, amusement, sadness, anxiety, or whatever, that belong to herself and her own life and are not in any way connected to either the supervisee or his work. It is when the supervisor experiences a response, either in the form of feelings, memories, thoughts or images that she cannot truthfully relate to her own personal or professional situation, that these responses become potentially useful to the supervisee. Useful questions that the supervisor can ask herself in order to assist this process can include:

- Am I feeling tired (or angry or sad or confused or whatever) because of what the supervisee is saying to me at the moment, or for some other reason?
- How do I feel, generally, about this supervisee?
- Do I always (or usually) feel tired (or angry or sad or confused, etc.) when speaking to this supervisee?
- Is there something particular in my life (either professional or personal) that is making me feel that at the moment?
- Is it possible that my current response has less to do with my general feelings about the supervisee, and about my own situation, and more to do with either how the supervisee or the patients are responding to the nursing care being described?

Typical issues   Because this 'eye' involves the use of the supervisor's own personal response to the supervision material it would be misleading to suggest particular issues that may arise. The supervisor will know when she is using this 'eye' if having considered the questions above, the feeling, memory, thought or image she had is still strong. It will be her decision then whether to share this with her supervisee or not. I would suggest that she

Think about . . . the six eyes of clinical supervision for nurses

1 Read each of the following six statements, made by a supervisor to her supervisee, and decide which supervision 'eye' the supervisor was using to 'view' the supervisee's nursing care when she made each statement.

(a) 'I was wondering what you said to Mr Brown after he told you that he was feeling more depressed?'

(b) 'Would you be able to tell me something about Mr Brown's nursing history, from before he was last referred to you?'

(c) 'Can you say what it is that you think Mr Brown expects from you as his named nurse?'

(d) 'As you were telling me about how calm Mr Brown sounded when he told you about his difficulties, I suddenly had a mental image of a time-bomb ticking away.'

(e) 'I wonder how it feels for you to talk about the last time you met Mr Brown, right now?'

(f) 'For some time now, you have been saying that you would prefer it if I told you what to do about Mr Brown. I wonder if Mr Brown thinks that you should be more directive with him, too?'

2 The list below contains a range of supervisory tasks that a supervisor may undertake during the course of a typical supervision. For each task below:

(i) state which clinical supervision 'eye' that you expect her to be using to think about the task.

(ii) suggest a statement or question – in keeping with the 'eye' you have chosen – that the supervisor might use in order to complete her task in the most satisfactory way.

(a) The supervisor wishes to assist the supervisee to express his feelings about a particular situation he has described concerning his nursing care of Mr Brown.

(b) The supervisor wishes to assist the supervisee in designing a nursing care plan most suitable for Mr Brown.

(c) The supervisor wishes to have the supervisee consider alternative nursing strategies to the ones he has described using with Mr Brown.

(d) The supervisor wishes to allow the supervisee to consider any potential connection between his nursing care of Mr Brown and his clinical supervision.

(e) The supervisor wishes to offer the supervisee a new way of thinking about his nursing care of Mr Brown, through the use of a memory from her own nursing experience.

(f) The supervisor wishes to use the 'helicopter view' or 'fly-on-the-wall' style of supervision to help the supervisee to better understand the nature of the nursing relationship he is having with Mr Brown.

Table 6.8   *Samples Box 6 – the sixth 'eye' of clinical supervision*

The sixth 'eye' of clinical supervision – the supervisor's response to the supervision material

The supervisor's intention	Sample meta-questions
A To offer the supervisee a comment based upon a hunch, intuition, gut feeling or educated guess that she has about the supervisee's work.	1 'As I was listening to you describe Mr Brown's relationship with his wife I suddenly began to wonder if he had been married before.' 2 'I can't remember if you said that Mr Brown had been married before, or perhaps that's just how it seems to me from what you have been saying about his relationship with his wife.'
B To offer the supervisee a comment based upon recalled memories and/ or thoughts relating either to her work with this supervisee, other supervisees or her own clinical work.	1 'As you were describing Mr Brown, I got a memory flash about someone else I knew of with similar difficulties. I remember with that person, that his problems became considerably worse, for a short while, until he became reconciled to his divorce.'
C To offer the supervisee a comment based upon a sudden and otherwise inexplicable emotional reaction in the supervisor.	1 'I have started to feel quite angry listening to you speak of Mr Brown's relationship with his wife. Although you haven't mentioned anger, I do wonder if that has anything to do with how he may be feeling?' 2 'Although you told me that Mr Brown said that he fully understood the medical reasons for his treatment, I have started to feel a little perturbed while listening to you talk of him. Is it possible that, deep, down, he could be feeling worried too?' 3 'You said that when Mr Brown had separated from his wife, just before he was admitted to hospital, he had felt it was the best thing to happen, under the circumstances. I wonder why, then, I am feeling so sad when I listen to you talk about it?' 4 'When you were describing how Mr Brown was admitted to hospital immediately after being separated from his wife, I suddenly started to think about Daniel going into the lion's den.'

does this tentatively and carefully and in such a way that the supervisee is aware that he can reject the suggestion if it is not one that makes immediate sense to him. It would therefore be sensible for the supervisor to begin offering her response with a phrase such as:

- 'this may mean nothing to you but, while you were speaking I had a sudden memory of . . .'
- 'I am not sure if this will make any sense to you, but what you were saying reminded me of . . .'
- 'I suddenly got a picture of . . . in my mind, does that mean anything to you?'

Table 6.8 gives possible reasons for use of the 'supervisor's response eye' and samples of the types of statements (meta-questions) that the supervisor might make to her supervisee when discussing the supervisee's work in this category.

7

The Middle Phase of Supervision – Power, Persecution and Game-Playing

Key issues in this chapter

- The middle phase of clinical supervision
- Problems associated with the supervisee's development
- Dealing with anger and apathy in supervision
- Forms of power in clinical supervision
- The persecutory supervisor
- Game-playing in supervision

The middle phase of clinical supervision – progress and problems

The middle phase of supervision cannot be easily determined, in terms of weeks or months, because the total duration of the supervision will be unknown, in most cases, until it is over. What I am referring to, then, is more easily understood as a sense of 'being-together', shared by the supervisor and her supervisee, that has gone beyond the initial 'getting to know each other' stage. The supervisor will have become more familiar with the work of her supervisee and they will both have begun to relax in each other's company. The supervisee may even have left behind some of the anxiety that he originally attached to being in the company of his supervisor. Perhaps the most obvious sign that the supervision has reached its 'middle-phase' is that both the supervisor and her supervisee will have begun to feel comfortable and settled both with the supervision work, and with each other. Although this development will be welcomed by many, it can also have its potential drawbacks for the supervision work and the professional relationship between the supervisor and her supervisee. In this section I will discuss some possible reasons why this might occur and offer suggestions on how to deal with the more detrimental aspects of clinical supervision.

The 'middle phase' of clinical supervision is not dissimilar to the middle phase of a marriage or long-term relationship. The novelty and excitement found in the early stages of the liaison may have passed, and the partners are settling down to a possibly less exciting – but potentially no less valid and interesting – time together. The danger is, whether in marriage or supervision, that this period of settlement could be misunderstood as 'pointless' or 'boring' and ultimately work against the partners.

As with a marriage, the responsibility for problems and difficulties does not necessarily reside with one partner in isolation, and the supervisor is not free from the prospect of becoming apathetic and disinterested in her supervisee. This phase of the supervisory relationship is the one in which the supervisee will need to be most vigilant in her responses to her supervisee as there may be a tendency to switch off from what the supervisee is doing and saying. Again, as with a marriage, the more that the partners are aware of the dangers in advance, the better placed they will be to take preventative counter-action.

The fourth and fifth stages of a supervisee's development

DEVELOPMENT STAGE 4 – EXUBERANCE AND TAKING CHARGE

Friedman and Kaslow (1986) suggest that the fourth stage of the supervisee's professional development is one in which he begins to accept that he is professionally credible and, perhaps, that he has a professional mind of his own. He will begin to make more of his own connections between theory and practice, and to use his own reading and learning to inform his nursing work with patients.

Some nursing supervisees may also begin to express preferences for certain nursing models and theories or choose specific ways of working with patients over others. At this stage some supervisees might even consider specific, post-registration training in a method of nursing care that they perceive as most relevant to their work, and their own style of working. It is likely, in any event, that the supervisor will find herself on the receiving-end of the supervisee's self-generated knowledge and beliefs about what is best for his patients. Although the supervisee may still rely on his supervisor, the sense of 'not-knowing' and needing to be 'instructed' will probably diminish as the supervisee begins to see his supervisor as more of a 'consultant' or 'expert colleague', than a teacher. The supervisee at this stage of development will be ready for greater challenges in his nursing work and will be expressing a desire to move on professionally.

Potential problems of the supervisee's development
DEVELOPMENT STAGE 5 – IDENTITY AND INDEPENDENCE
The emergence of the clinical nurse supervisee into a fully-fledged and autonomous practitioner is not without its difficulties. Friedman and Kaslow (1986) have described the fifth stage of professional development as, the 'stage of professional adolescence'. If the supervisee is to become disillusioned, apathetic and conflictual towards his clinical supervisor and the supervision, then it is most likely to be during this stage of his development in clinical supervision. The supervisee's increasing sense of 'professional identity', coupled with his increasing knowledge and decreasing dependency on his supervisor, may result in him expressing differences of opinion and challenging the supervisor's views more often. He will feel safer about rejecting his supervisor's suggestions and even begin to see himself – sometimes justifiably – as more knowledgeable or 'expert' than his supervisor in some areas of nursing.

The emergence of anger and apathy
Moving onward and upward in terms of professional development is not unlike moving into adulthood for other reasons than described above. Parents may appear less attentive and less supportive to the adolescent child and the sense of being totally looked after fades, as the emergent-adult is increasingly expected to fend for himself. The clinical supervisee at this stage of his development can become angry with his supervisor who is seen to be no longer giving him all of the answers he needs, to solve the nursing problems he is facing in his everyday working life. The supervisee can be become angry and disillusioned with the supervisor for not providing his every supervisory need, although

this will often clash with his need to 'do his own thing'.

The clinical nurse supervisor should be prepared for a considerable amount of disillusionment being expressed by the supervisee about his experience of clinical supervision, and its value to himself specifically and the nursing profession generally. Some of this feedback may reach the supervisor and it should not be ignored or 'brushed under the carpet' but be treated like any other supervisory topic and discussed rationally and as objectively as possible. The problem may be complicated – and potentially compounded – if the supervisor hears complaints or expressions of supervisee dissatisfaction from a third party.

Avoiding apathy

Some suggestions for avoiding apathy in clinical nursing supervision include:

MAKE VARIETY THE SPICE OF SUPERVISORY LIFE
- If the supervisee brings more than one patient each session, change the order of presentation, and perhaps the time allowed for presentation.
- Try different supervisory techniques – but not at the risk of becoming out of your depth or providing inadequate input.
- It is a perfectly valid educational technique to cover old material at a different level or depth. Try using the *six-eyes* model to bring the supervisee to a different level of understanding of the same issue. It is one thing for him to understand the content of the patient's problem and a completely different one for him to understand his own emotional response to it.

IF YOU FEEL 'STUCK', MOVE ON
Do not dwell on a problem that threatens to linger and dominate the process. Move on to new areas of the supervisee's work and come back to the source of his 'stuckness' later.

Think about this . . . avoiding the apathy

1 Bring to mind any long term, one-to-one relationship – personal or professional – that became boring or uninteresting for you at times.
2 Make two lists. One (list A) of the feelings that you had during the boring times and another (list B) of the feelings that these replaced, that were prevalent at the beginning of the relationship.

3 Think about why the feelings in list B went away. What was it about
   the relationship – and your part in it – that caused the excitement to
   lessen and the apathy to increase?
4 What could you have done to have kept the relationship fresh and to
   prevent the onset of boredom?

Forms of power in clinical supervision

An important concept in clinical supervision is the notion of
power. Morrall (1985) states that: 'Power exists when an
individual behaves in such a way that it will produce a change
in another individual.' It would follow that the clinical nurse
supervisor is in a position to exert much power over her
supervisee, should she choose to do so. Even when power is not
being exerted consciously, the supervisor needs to be aware how
her actions may inadvertently cause her to put the supervisee in a
powerless position.

McQuail (1984) has indicated a number of ways in which power
can be exploited through communication and I have adapted
these to clinical supervision for nurses. The clinical nurse
supervisor would gain from becoming alert to the potential of
exerting power in some of the following detrimental ways:

MONOPOLISING THE CONVERSATION
This can have the effect of gaining control and achieving a desired
outcome. If the supervisory dominance goes unchallenged it is
likely that the supervisor will gain more control over the situation
and continue to dominate in a negative cycle.

POWER THROUGH CREDIBILITY
The clinical supervisor may take advantage of her elevated status
and professional credibility to unfairly influence, and take
advantage of the supervisee.

THE POWER OF IGNORANCE
Similarly, the clinical supervisor may take advantage of her status
and increased knowledge to influence the supervisee with inaccurate or ill-informed information. The supervisee may decide not
to challenge such erroneous messages in view of his perceived

inferior and/or less knowledgeable position in relation to his supervisor.

Morrall (1995) describes a range of different forms of power and I have, below, suggested some ways in which they might appear in the clinical supervision setting.

EXPERT POWER

'Expert' power can be exerted when one person assumes that another has greater knowledge and skills than themselves, perhaps as a result of extensive training or experience. It is feasible that the notion of 'expert' power could have great relevance within the clinical supervision setting. Even when clinical nurse supervisors wish to see themselves as equal in status to their supervisees and have no particular desire to exercise their authority or control, it is possible that they might find themselves unwillingly thrust into the position of 'reluctant guru' by virtue of their 'expert power'. It might then become easier to exert control and influence – albeit unintentionally – over a supervisee who may have come to see his clinical supervisor as increasingly omnipotent, with a commensurate increase in her authority.

COERCIVE POWER

Coercive power exists when one individual can exert 'punishment' over another. In the family situation, a typical example of coercive power might be the mother of a unruly child telling her to 'behave or I will send you to bed without your supper'. In the work situation, most senior – and middle – managers will be familiar with asking a subordinate to complete a task, in the knowledge that if they do not, a formal reprimand could – if not necessarily will – follow. As nurses, we may do what is expected of us because we enjoy the work and are committed to it. However, most of us also realise that if we were to persistently refuse reasonable requests to carry out the tasks for which we are employed – or act in a way that was contrary to our contract – then we could expect our seniors to exert 'coercive power' and discipline, or 'punish' us. The prospect of punishment through the use of coercion is unlikely to be a reality in the clinical supervision setting, where supervision of subordinates by managers is not advisable. It is not unknown, however, for supervisors to influence their supervisees through the covert assumption that they could exert coercive power – perhaps through the unfair influence of other professionals and senior colleagues, should they wish to do so. It is important that the supervisor closely monitors her input for the possibility that she might, even inadvertently, threaten her supervisee with the suggestion that she might use her managerial connections to his detriment.

REWARD POWER
'Reward power' can be exerted where an individual has the ability to reward another either by providing positive elements or by removing negative ones. Again, because of the lack of managerial influence in the supervision relationship, it seems unlikely that the clinical nurse supervisor would be in a position to control the supervisee's behaviour, with the use of a psychological – or practical – 'reward and forfeit' system. The conditions for such subtle control will be determined by the precise nature of the professional relationship that exists between supervisor and supervisee outside the supervision situation.

LEGITIMATE POWER
The concept of 'legitimate power' applies where it is accepted that a person has the right and authority – usually of society or an organisation – to have influence and control over others (e.g. a magistrate, police officer or the head of an organisation or department – including the nurse-manager of a ward). It is a matter of some debate whether the notion of 'legitimate power' can be appropriately applied to the clinical supervision situation. If it is accepted that the clinical supervisor is not managerially responsible for, or hierarchically superior to, the supervisee, then it should follow that power cannot be exerted over the supervisee in the 'legitimate' sense. Any assertions that the supervisee may make in defence of his behaviour or actions to the effect: 'I did it because my supervisor suggested it/told me to/would approve ... etc.', might be more correctly associated with the influence of 'expert' or 'coercive' power than its 'legitimate' form. Supervisors and their supervisees need to remain alert to the potential to confuse the supervisory function – which should not afford the clinical nurse supervisor with 'legitimate power' in the true sense – with a managerial or hierarchical relationship, which will usually allow for the exertion, appropriately or otherwise, of this form of authority.

REFERENT POWER
The influence of 'referent power' operates in conditions where one person has attributes that another wishes he had, who then

identifies with, and possibly tries to emulate, that person in order that he, too, becomes 'powerful'. Whether they try to avoid it or not, many clinical supervisors will be the subject of identification and emulation by their supervisees. This is understandable, to some extent, because most beginners, in whatever field, will benefit from the learning they can glean from exposure to the skills, knowledge and experiences of an appropriate role-model. Clinical nurse supervisors should not be surprised to hear supervisees using similar words, phrases and even general speech patterns to their own. Depending on the level to which 'referent power' is being exerted, supervisees may begin to adopt body postures that they have observed in their supervisor, and even begin to dress in a similar manner. Clinical supervisees may initially look for a psychological 'peg' on to which they can, eventually, hang their own particular nursing 'hat', in terms of developing a style of thinking and behaving that they can call their own. Supervisors should therefore not be unduly concerned about being imitated, at least in the early stages of clinical supervision, assuming that they are satisfied that the thoughts and actions being emulated are clinically sound. 'Referent power' can begin to have a detrimental influence on the supervisee if he is not encouraged to eventually develop a style of his own, but instead becomes nothing more than a 'clone' of his clinical nurse supervisor.

INFORMATIONAL POWER

'Knowledge is power' is the often too-frequent, and anxiety-ridden, subtext in many hierarchical organisations. It suggests that control is maintained through the withholding of information or knowledge by one person who is privy to that information, from another person who is not. A connected assumption is that for as long as the knowledge-holder is choosing not to dis-seminate the information (usually to subordinates) she holds an advantage over these people and can exploit this for her own gain (or that of the organisation) and at the expense of the junior colleagues. Clinical nurse supervisors will frequently have – or be expected to have – more knowledge on certain matters than their supervisees. The real question for supervisors is not whether there is a knowledge-differential but, rather, how they deal with it, in relation to their supervisee. If both supervisor and supervisee can accept that there is an imbalance with regard to their respective experiences and knowledge, this differential can be applied in a positive way to enhance the supervisory relationship and the supervisee's clinical development.

Think about . . . power in relationships

1 Think about some of the relationships that you have and list two or three of the people you are most closely involved with, in each of the following situations:
   a) At home
   b) At work
   c) Socially.
2 By each name, write down some requests, demands or wishes that they have expressed and which you have acted upon, recently.
3 Think about what it is that motivates you to act on the requests and wishes of those people. What particular form of power – if any – is being exerted over you by those people? Are these requests/wishes/demands always valid and appropriate? Do you ever act against your better judgement? If so, are you acting in response to the exertion of a particular form of power?

The persecutory supervisor

The experience of clinical supervision can be one of the most enlightening and rewarding times in a nurse's professional life. It can offer new insights, new ways of working and an opportunity to discuss troublesome issues that is unparalleled.

However the position of clinical supervisor – with its inherent notion of power and superior knowledge – automatically grants its holder a potential to harm and irrevocably damage the supervisee. Even if the supervisor has no intention of abusing her privileged position – and I suggest, carefully, that the *majority* of supervisors do not set out with that intention – the potential to do so, under the circumstances, is unfortunately still great.

Meares and Hobson (1977), discussing the problems incurred when practising psychoanalytic psychotherapy, outlined six main categories of types of behaviour, by the therapist, that can result in the patient feeling worse instead of better – or *persecuted*. While I am not suggesting that the work of a clinical nurse supervisor is, or should be, akin to that of a psychotherapist, I do believe that there are certain parallels, here, in terms of the sort of unhelpful and potentially divisive comments and behaviours that both of these health professionals can offer.

The clinical nurse supervisor needs to monitor her intervention style constantly to ensure that it remains one that the supervisee considers positive and helpful. Many supervisors would be surprised to learn that what they have to say is considered negative and even destructive and times. But if the supervisee is new, inexperienced, especially anxious and/or unsure of the supervisor then this is a perfectly feasible outcome, even if the supervisory comment is intended to be, at best, constructive or, at least, innocuous.

The six categories of persecution outlined by Meares and Hobson (1997) are listed below, with my suggestions on how they may present themselves in clinical nursing supervision.

INTRUSION

The supervisor acts like a prosecuting counsel and demands that the supervisee defends himself in terms of his actions and behaviours. 'Why did you do that?' and 'What were you thinking of . . .?' are common questions in the intrusive supervisor's repertoire. Her questions will be probing and her tone of voice sharp. There is an underlying suggestion that the supervisee needs to answer all of the questions put to him – a bit like being in the dock, in court. The more anxious the supervisor becomes, the more likely she is to become *intrusive*. This can be one of the most potentially damaging forms of persecution in supervision. Should this situation continue for any length of time the supervisory relationship may fail to recover from it.

DEROGATION

The derogatory supervisor makes her supervisee feel bad and worthless, lowers his self-esteem and encourages his sense of guilt about being not as good as she is. The derogatory supervisor does not attempt to disguise her view that she knows best and is much more experienced than the supervisee. Common phrases for her to use would include 'It's so long since I've made those mistakes . . .', 'I can't remember ever doing that, but I'll try to help', 'It sounds like you've got yourself into a serious mess'. The supervisee will be left feeling afraid to expose himself and his difficulties for fear of being ridiculed.

INVALIDATION OF EXPERIENCE

When the clinical nurse supervisor tells her supervisee that he does not really mean what he is saying, she is invalidating his experience. It is a form of attack, according to Meares and Hobson (1977), that is more subtle than those of intrusion and derogation but no less damaging. A common way for supervisors to do this is to pick up on technical jargon and replace the supervisee's own language with the 'correct' usage. More damaging still, is the supervisor's insistence that something did not actually happen in the way that the supervisee described it, for example, 'That patient could not possibly have broken his foot, it must have been a severe sprain.' In an extreme case, the supervisor will insist that her supervisee does not know his own mind by suggesting that his emotional response to the nursing situation being described, is inaccurate: 'Surely that would not make you angry, but I can see how you would become frustrated.'

THE OPAQUE SUPERVISOR

Everyone likes feedback. A supervisee needs to know if he is on the right lines and – probably even more importantly – that what he has to say has registered with the supervisor on some emotional level. He needs to know that his supervisor is interested, that she finds his work intriguing, enjoyable to listen to, frustrating or challenging. Whatever the supervisory response may be it is preferable to no response at all. The phrase *opaque supervisor* is used to describe someone that cannot be seen through, emotionally. It is a supervisor who remains totally neutral and emotionally unresponsive to whatever she is told, thus giving the hapless supervisee no encouragement – or even discouragement – to continue with what he has to say. She is also unlikely to answer any questions or offer advice other than by saying something like 'what would you like to do about it?'

UNTENABLE SITUATIONS

The concept of the 'untenable situation' suggests any occurrence during the supervisee's experience of supervision that causes him to feel 'stuck' or disadvantaged and unable to respond to his supervisor in a way that allows him to feel that he is benefiting from supervision. When a supervisee finds himself in an 'untenable situation', his first response may be to leave both the room, immediately, and the supervisory experience, permanently. It is worth noting that clinical nurse supervisors should do whatever they can to avoid the occurrence of such a situation because, even if the supervisee is able to recover from it sufficiently to maintain his trust in his supervisor and also his determination to continue to be supervised by her, some damage will inevitably be done to their professional relationship. Below I offer four main ways in which the untenable situation can occur in clinical supervision for nurses, based on the original work of Meares and Hobson (1977).

The untenable structures of supervision   Although it may seem obvious, the supervisee needs to know what he is expected to do. If there is no structure to supervision then it will be difficult for him to know when to start speaking and when to stop. In a boundaryless supervision the supervisee will simply become stuck and unable to function.

The untenable demands by supervisors   Supervisors must recognise that the supervisees will function at different levels. Some may require much coaxing and guidance to express themselves and their situations fully, while others may simply need a 'go on . . .' from the supervisor to spark off their thought processes. Supervisors must be sensitive to what they can offer to best encourage their supervisee to express himself fully and accurately. An intervention suitable for an experienced supervisee may prove to be an impossible demand for a beginner.

A supervisor who tells her supervisee to say more about the situation he is discussing, while in a tone of voice that expresses a sense of total boredom will cause him to feel confused about what he is really meant to do and he will be ultimately stuck and unable to do anything. Similarly, if the supervisor has expressed her dislike of a particular kind of patient or situation previously, the supervisee, even though desperate to raise an issue of a similar nature, may want to protect his supervisor from the material and, again, the unsatisfactory result will be that he does nothing. Learning how to adjust communication styles in order to relate to different types of supervisees, in different situations can be one way of alleviating the problem of untenable demands on the supervisee.

The untenable messages of supervisors   The supervisor must be alert to the notion that she can say one thing in words and something quite different by the tone of her voice, gestures, facial expressions and other non-verbal communication. Hobson and Meares (1977) suggest that this 'double-talk' is likely to lead to feelings of uncertainty, perplexity, confusion and persecution in the supervisee. It is important that the supervisor is consistent in her message. If she is pleased she should look it, as well as say it. If she is angry or frustrated or wishing to express any negative emotion in relation to the supervisee's material she should never do this through a false smile or even neutral expression. The more that the supervisor can learn to express herself with honesty and integrity, the safer and more trusting her supervisee will become.

The vicious circle of supervision   Once the supervisee has begun to experience supervision in a negative way it is likely that this will quickly increase and at worst become unbearable, causing him to drop out unless it is dealt with by the supervisor. Perhaps surprisingly a major factor in the exacerbation of this destructive force will be the level in which the supervisor is likely to feel persecuted herself, by the supervisee. Meares and Hobson (1977) suggest that owing to her own personality structure and current problems, the supervisee is not alone in experiencing various forms of being 'got at'. The supervisor can also experience the supervisee as being intolerably intrusive, derogatory, opaque and inconsistent. As with any human being, the extent to which this is experienced – and her response to it – will depend on her personality structure and level of self-awareness. At worst, the supervisor will attack the supervisee, either overtly or covertly by use of subtle means and game-playing.

Game-playing in supervision

Many nurses will be familiar with the work of Eric Berne who, in his book *Games People Play* (1964), introduced the notion that human beings employ various schemes or *games* which are designed specifically for the purpose of helping them meet some personal objective or goal.

Berne defined a game as 'an on-going series of complementary ulterior transactions – superficially plausible but with a concealed motivation'. The whole purpose of a game is that it should pro-duce the desired purpose or goal for the person instigating it quickly and easily, and usually allow them to reduce the level of threat or pain – often perceived psychologically if not physically – that they are experiencing, or feel that they could experience, in their present situation.

Although Berne proposed that game-playing is very common in everyday life, another writer, Alfred Kadushin, has applied

Berne's principles to the practice of clinical supervision. Although originally outlined in 1968, with social workers in mind, Kadushin's concepts of game-playing in clinical supervision are still relevant, and I have adapted his original theories to the process of clinical nurse supervision.

The main purpose of games in supervision, according to Kadushin, is to protect the supervisee from the many threats presented to him by being in supervision. As I have discussed in Chapter 5, it is possible that the supervisee will feel disadvantaged and insecure as a consequence of receiving clinical supervision. If this is the case, it is a natural response for him to want to keep some sense of control over the situation, which he may feel he can do by playing a psychological game with his supervisor.

Kadushin grouped the types of games that supervisees play into various sections that define their particular purpose. I have offered my own version of Kadushin's main groupings below together with my adaptation of the specific games that can be used in each group to help the supervisee reduce his level of anxiety and threat.

GAMES TO MANIPULATE DEMAND LEVELS
There are a whole series of games specifically designed to help the supervisee manipulate the level of demand made on him, by the organisation or his work generally. Many nursing supervisees, particularly those who are more interested in the practical 'hands on' aspects of the job, are likely to become impatient and frustrated with routine procedures. Newly qualified nurses may, for example, be very good at carrying out complex physical procedures to a very high standard, but be less adept at writing this procedure up properly in the case notes or recording it and reporting it in some other routine manner.

Supervisee Game 1: 'Me And You Against The Trust': The following scenario is an example of one such game aimed at manipulating the demand levels on the supervisee.

> *Supervisee*: Sometimes I think that my charge nurse has got something against me. I am working really hard at the moment, and developing a good many skills and yet she never seems to be satisfied. Take yesterday, for example, my clinical work couldn't be faulted. I carried out some nursing procedures that even she would be proud of, and everyone in my care, and most of my other colleagues seemed to think I was doing a really good practical job. But what did the charge

nurse say at the end of the day? Only: 'Well you've done the work but you haven't written-up the notes properly'! Really – is that being picky or what?

Supervisor: And had you written up the notes properly?

Supervisee: Well, no actually, I hadn't. But I was so busy doing the work that I hadn't got time and, anyway, it's not really what clinical nurses should be doing is it? I mean, you know that as well as anyone, you're a very skilled clinical nurse yourself. I am *sure* that you must sympathise with my predicament!

Supervisor: I am not clear exactly what predicament you are in; other than having no time to complete your work by writing it up in the notes?

Supervisee: I thought you might say that. I can see that you understand my situation, but it's not really your position to say that you do, is it? I mean, any highly-skilled clinical nurse would surely disagree with the idea that we have to waste our time filling in useless pieces of paper rather than getting on with what we are good at – nursing the people in our care!

It is now the supervisor, rather than her supervisee who could be in a predicament. It is quite feasible that the supervisee has expressed a view that she is only too familiar with and with which she may, indeed, have some sympathy. On the other hand, it is clear that the supervisee is not carrying out her role fully since in failing to do the proper paperwork she is not completing her tasks.

So far, however, the supervisor is on reasonably safe ground. Although the supervisee has introduced the notion of playing the game 'Me and You Against the Trust' it takes two to play any game, and the supervisor has yet to be induced. Game-playing of this nature is never positive and the supervisor must ensure that she is not drawn into colluding with the supervisee against the demands he feels are being put upon him by the charge nurse and ultimately the nursing organisation for which he works. It is very likely that the supervisee has already said things that the supervisor is able to relate to, including the concern of nurses that too much time is spent on paperwork and not enough time is spent exercising clinical skills. The supervisor may accept that the supervisee has read her correctly in assuming that she is also someone with concerns about this situation. It is possible, too, that a new supervisor may find difficulty in asserting her view against the supervisee for fear that this may unfavourably affect the supervisory relationship.

Although the supervisor must give serious thought to the reasons why she may want to play this game, it is essential that she does not allow herself to be enticed. The supervisor's task, here, is to find some way of showing the supervisee that he is attempting to encourage his supervisor to collude with him in an allegiance against his charge nurse, the nursing organisation, and the existing conditions under which he currently works. It would be more conducive to his professional development if the supervisor were able to encourage her supervisee to discuss some of the difficulties he faces in working under such conditions. She might also wish to explore some of the strategies he might employ to help him deal with them.

Supervisee Game 2: 'Be As Good to Me As I Am to You': This is another game designed to control the level of demand made upon the nursing supervisee and one in which he sets out to seduce his supervisor through flattery. The chief ploy in this game is for the supervisee to spend a good deal of time telling the supervisor how wonderful she is. Phrases like: 'You are the best supervisor I have ever had', 'You're so intuitive and receptive it is almost as if you can read my mind', 'I have never found anyone that is so consistently helpful' and 'Everything you say makes complete sense to me' will trip off the supervisee's tongue with such regularity and deftness that the supervisor may secretly conclude that her once-reticent supervisee has enrolled in a charm-school course at the week-ends.

Even the most seasoned and hard-bitten supervisor will find it hard not to succumb to such a barrage of consistent flattery. It is possible, of course, that the supervisee means every word that he says. There is no reason to suspect that just because a supervisee is flattering and kind towards his supervisor that his intentions are sinister and that there is an ulterior motive behind his praise. Whatever the reason for the flattery, however, the supervisor needs to guard against the danger of allowing herself to become blinded by it. If this happens, she may find it difficult to resist requests – however subtle – to support the supervisee in a stand against the organisation or other colleagues with whom he works and is having difficulty.

An important – and, in my view, entirely reasonable – source of gratification for the supervisor is that which she receives through helping her supervisee to grow and develop as a nurse. In order to do this, it may be necessary for the supervisor to glean at least some information from the supervisee about how good a job she is doing. The task for the supervisor here is to avoid becoming so interested in and overwhelmed by any praise she may receive from her supervisee, that she allows it to affect her objective judgement of his work and to remain reasonably detached in her role.

GAMES TO REDEFINE THE SUPERVISORY RELATIONSHIP

This second set of games also has the fundamental purpose of reducing the level of professional demands made on the nursing supervisee. The main difference is that, in the first group of games the supervisee sets out to encourage his supervisor to collude with him against the organisation – although the nature of the supervisor–supervisee relationship remains intact. In this set of games the main aim is to reduce the pressure on the supervisee through bringing about a fundamental change in the nature of the supervisory relationship itself.

These games will be easier to play for the supervisee if the relationship between himself and his supervisor is not clearly defined from the start. The more that the supervisor can do to define the boundaries and limits of the supervisory relationship, as described in Chapter 5, the more difficult it will be for the supervisee to start to play this game at all.

Supervisee Game 3: 'If You Were My Friend You Would Not Judge Me': The purpose of this game is for the supervisee to redefine the supervision relationship as a friendship. There are many different ways in which this game can be played, some subtle and some not-so-subtle. It is important that the supervisee does what he can to ingratiate himself with the supervisor, and the more inventive he can be on this matter, the more chance he may have of winning the game. I have offered, below, some ploys that newer players of this game could consider, but clinical nurse supervisors need to be aware that expert players are renowned for the subtlety and inventiveness of their ploys, which can be almost undetectable to all but the very alert.

The supervisee may arrange to take his lunch breaks at the same time as his supervisor and engage in friendly chat about the latest film or an interesting TV programme; he may 'accidentally' meet the supervisor in the local supermarket and engage in a discussion about the soaring price of potatoes; arrive at the clinical supervision with details of a particular conference or lecture which he feels would be of interest to both of them; bring to supervision books, videos or other material which he may consider to be of interest to the supervisor on a personal level and any number of other subtle ploys to encourage his supervisor to feel more like a friend towards him than a professional colleague.

The task for the supervisor is to try to maintain a friendly approach to her delivery of supervision without necessarily crossing the boundary from supervisor to friend. Friends, on the whole, are more easily coerced or manipulated than colleagues. It is much harder for the supervisor who is a friend of her supervisee to decline a request and much easier for her to conspire with him against the organisation, than it would be from the position of objective colleague.

One of the hardest tasks for the supervisor to accomplish is achieving the finely balanced position of what I like to refer to as *friendly objectivity*. This is a notion close to Hobson's (1985) 'aloneness-togetherness', which I have outlined in Chapter 5. 'Friendly objectivity' is not an easy state for any clinical supervisor to reach with her supervisee. It involves regular scrutiny of professional boundaries by the supervisor while, at the same time, she ensures that her demeanour and attitude towards her supervisee is always *genuinely* attentive, caring and generous. A good starting point for achieving this is if the supervisor determines never to take on anyone that she knows socially as a supervisee. Similarly, and possibly more importantly, the clinical nurse supervisor should never agree to a social relationship with anyone she is currently supervising. When those rules are firmly in place it will be easier to be positively disposed towards the supervisee – even to like him – without fearing that this will lead the supervisor to collude with or be manipulated by her supervisee.

GAMES TO REDUCE THE SUPERVISOR'S POWER

Even though clinical nursing supervision is not about the hier-archical judgement or management of a junior colleague by a more senior one it will be very difficult for the supervisee, particularly at the beginning stages of his supervisory experience, to not feel that his supervisor is more powerful than he is, and has more influence and control than he does. Although the clinical nurse supervisor should not have managerial power or links to management which may cause the supervisee anxiety, she will still be regarded as more powerful by virtue of her expertise, greater knowledge and superior clinical skills. The supervisee's main goal is to reduce his level of threat – and quite possibly a sense of being deskilled – by playing a game which will allow him to feel that the supervisor is not quite so clever after all.

Supervisee Game 4: 'If You Knew Nightingale Like I Know Nightingale':
A typical version of this game would be played as outlined in the
scenario below.

> *Supervisee*: I was thinking about what happened last time we met, when
> I was describing my nursing care of Mr Brown. It has occurred to me
> that I am employing completely the wrong model of nursing care for
> someone with his clinical requirements.
>
> *Supervisor*: Really?
>
> *Supervisee*: Yes. Actually, I am a bit surprised that you didn't mention it
> yourself. I read only last week in *The International Journal of Super-
> Nursing* about a revision of the Rawles-Bentley nursing model,
> which now incorporates a unique blend of the original thinking with
> new theories derived from Quantum Physics. I suppose you didn't
> want to mention it to me until I was a little more advanced in my
> professional development.
>
> *Supervisor*: [*feeling confused*] Er . . . I . . . erm . . . oh, yes . . . I suppose
> that's the reason. Remind me of that model's basic principles, will
> you, just to make sure that we're both on the same wave length
> about it.
>
> *Supervisee*: [*feeling smug*] Certainly. Well, the main points are that . . .

It is equally clear to both parties that the supervisor has never
heard of the Rawles-Bentley model nor its revised amalgamation
with Quantum Physics. Her fumbled response to the supervisee's
statement that he has spotted this new and apparently superior
way of thinking, has simply underlined this fact and helped the
supervisee to feel even more that he has scored some valuable
points over his supervisor. At the point that the supervisee pro-
ceeds to instruct his supervisor about the new model, the implicit
roles of teacher–learner are suddenly reversed. The supervisee
is then able to feel, at least to some extent, that the power disparity between them is reduced, and with it the supervisee's
perceived level of inadequacy in relation to his more experienced
supervisor.

The game of 'If You Knew Nightingale Like I Know Nightingale' only works if the supervisor refuses to accept that she is
totally ignorant to what the supervisee is referring. Likewise, the
supervisee does not openly expose his supervisor nor condemn
her as ignorant and compounds the problem. The game only
really works well if both parties 'pretend' that they both know
what they are talking about. The problem for the supervisor is that
she is left feeling, at best, guilty and depressed about the notion
that she knows less than her supervisee and that she has been

afraid to say so. Ultimately, there is nothing wrong with allowing the supervisee to feel that the power disparity between them has been reduced.

When clinical nurse supervision is working well it will be devoid of power struggles. The more that the supervisor can do to allow her supervisee to feel less like an ignorant child and more like a willing collaborator towards the goal of enhanced nursing skills and knowledge, the easier it will be for both parties to work towards that aim. The supervisor's task, when this game is recognised, is to accept that so long as the supervisee is attending he must feel that there is still more to gain from the professional relationship. The more that the supervisor can accept this notion, the less afraid she should become to admitting to gaps in her knowledge or experience.

GAMES PLAYED TO CONTROL SUPERVISION

This set of games is mainly concerned with how the supervisee can shift control of the supervision situation from the clinical nurse supervisor to himself. Lack of control over the clinical supervision is potentially threatening to the supervisee because it may mean that his supervisor will take the initiative to introduce a discussion of issues that may highlight the supervisee's short-comings, weak spots and inadequacies. The supervisor may at no time consciously intend to raise anything that will deliberately cause her supervisee to feel inadequate, but in any learning situation a time is bound to arise when, in order for development to occur, the learner will need to address unfamiliar and challenging issues. Consequently, the more control that the nursing supervisee has over the supervision situation, the more he can use it to avoid talking about those things which will lead him to feel inadequate.

Supervisee Game 5: 'My Little List': The rules of the game are quite simple and are as follows:

1   The supervisee must arrive at the supervision session with a list of questions about his clinical nursing work – either in his head or written down – that he would very much like to discuss with the supervisor.
2   The supervisee will then ask his questions of his supervisor, beginning with those questions that he knows the supervisor has most knowledge of and interest in.

3   Question one having been asked, the supervisor begins a short
    lecture on the topic, giving as much information as possible
    and embellishing her answer with references from various
    nursing texts and perhaps using short anecdotes from her
    clinical career.
4   While the supervisor is delivering her short lecture, the super-
    visee is under no obligation to listen to what she is saying. The
    supervisee can, if he so wishes, think about anything else that
    may occur to him of either a personal or professional nature. It
    is important, however, that the supervisee remembers to nod
    occasionally at salient points during his supervisor's mono-
    logue, and to maintain an expression of fascinated interest on
    his face throughout.
5   At the conclusion of the first monologue, the supervisee must
    ask his second question. The game is then continued in a
    circular fashion, from point 2 (above).
6   The game is won if the supervisee continues to ask a series of
    questions to which he has no interest in the answers what-
    soever, until the end of the supervision session itself.
7   The game is lost if the supervisor is able, at some point during
    any monologue, to realise that she is being hoodwinked into
    time-wasting by the supervisee in order that the latter player
    can avoid discussion of issues or topics that he may find
    sensitive or challenging.

When the supervisee becomes particularly skilled at this game
he will make his list so that it begins with the topics that he knows
his supervisor is particularly familiar with and has the greatest
professional interest in. An important reason for the supervisor
becoming involved in this game, at all, is that she will gain some
personal pleasure in showing off her knowledge and consequently feeling helpful to the supervisee. There may also be an
implicit idea around for the supervisor that it is her role to answer
any and all questions that are asked of her by her supervisee, and
that if she does not do this she will be failing in her supervisory
duty. The task for the supervisor, here, is to discern when appropriate questions are being asked, and which ones should be
answered accordingly. The considerate supervisor will not wish
to do anything to make her supervisee feel insecure or threatened
by focusing the issues on him and his shortcomings, but she
should at the same time be conscious that in order for him to
move on he will sooner or later need to address sensitive issues.

GAMES PLAYED TO CREATE A PSYCHOLOGICAL 'DISTANCE'

The clinical nurse supervisee can also control the degree to which he feels threatened by supervision through the use of *distancing techniques*. He can choose to share information about his work in a way that does not offer the true picture of his professional activities – and his concerns about them – and which keeps the disclosure on a superficial level. He can choose to share information selectively and can even distort the information he gives to his supervisor – either wittingly or unwittingly – in order to present a more favourable picture of himself.

Supervisee Game 6: 'What You Don't Know Can't Hurt Me': This game is a typical example of one used as a distancing technique and also one that is likely to be played by most – if not all – clinical nurse supervisees at some point in their supervisory experience. The fact that this game can be played at all is due to a fundamental principle of clinical supervision: the supervisor has no control over exactly what her supervisee chooses to say to her. There is no real winner of this game because the supervisee will only gain from supervision in proportion to what he puts into it. The more that the supervisor can encourage, albeit carefully and gradually, the supervisee to disclose about his professional life at deeper and more potentially threatening levels, the more he is likely to feel that he is on the road to enhanced practice.

Think about . . . why supervisors allow game-playing

It is generally accepted that it takes two people to play a game – whether physical or psychological. With that in mind, consider the following questions:

1 For what reasons might you, as a clinical supervisor allow yourself to become embroiled in something that is by its nature unproductive, and which allows the supervisee to avoid addressing some of the more pertinent – if difficult – issues raised by the clinical supervision itself?
2 How might a supervisor be enticed into helping her supervisee avoid the difficult aspects of his nursing work, his personality and clinical supervision itself?
3 How easy would it be for you to join in the game-playing with a supervisee?
4 What situations or circumstances might increase the possibility for you to be drawn into game-playing with a supervisee?

Games that clinical nurse supervisors might play

The clinical nurse supervisor is not incapable of feeling threatened by the supervision situation, herself. It is feasible then that she may too wish to instigate certain games during the clinical supervision process that allow her to feel safer, less vulnerable, approved of by the supervisee, and in extreme cases to even exert some control or power over the supervisee. It is worth noting that some of the games described above, as ones that have particular benefit for the nurse-supervisee, can also be gainfully used by the supervisor, at any time she is feeling particularly insecure and in need of reassurance that she is as good as she hopes. 'If You Knew Nightingale Like I Know Nightingale' is an especially good example of a game that can be used equally to the benefit of both supervisor and supervisee, and could in extreme cases be alternated from one to the other.

Supervisor Game 1: 'Was that What You Really Meant to Say?': This game can be played by supervisors when they are trying to reassure themselves that their supervisee is not really as talented or as clever as he may seem. It is probably also likely to be played when the supervisor finds herself on the receiving end of a challenge to her knowledge-base from the supervisee. The most reasonable course of action in these cases may be for the supervisor to reassess her understanding, and accept that the supervisee has the clearer grasp of the issue being discussed. If, however, the supervisor feels that this will be too threatening to her position, she may prefer to play this game. Instead of simply agreeing that the supervisee does, in fact, have a greater understanding of the issue than herself, she responds with 'Was that what you *really* meant to say?' – or a similarly demoralising challenge. Expert players may also employ a tone of voice that simultaneously implies not only is the supervisee completely *wrong* in his assertion, but also that he has an ulterior – probably seditious – reason for making the statement in the first place! The supervisee is thereby put firmly in the position of feeling that he has to explain why he challenged his supervisor at all and that, like a naughty child, he should feel suitably guilty for questioning his 'elders' and 'betters'. The real task for the clinical nurse supervisor, in such a situation, is to avoid starting the game at all, by becoming more open to the idea that all supervisees, no matter how clinically inexperienced, may have understanding and knowledge to equal – if not surpass – her own.

Supervisor Game 2: 'One Good Question Deserves Another': This is a very useful game for those supervisors who feel that they should know all of the answers to all of the questions that their super-visee might ever ask them, but who are simultaneously unable to use the phrase 'I am sorry I do not know the answer to that question'!

The rules for this game are particularly easy to grasp and most supervisors can become reasonably adept at it from the very first session with little effort.

1   When her supervisee asks any question, the clinical nurse supervisor is to respond with the phrase, 'Well, I could answer that question but I would like to know what you think about it yourself.'
2   The clinical nurse supervisor then sits in silence and waits for her supervisee to work out the answer to his own question (in supervisory terms this can be described as 'facilitating professional growth and development').
3   While waiting for a reply, the clinical nurse supervisor does her level best to think of a suitable response, in the event that her supervisee will be dumbfounded.

The usual outcome of this game is that the supervisee will offer an answer to his own question that may be wholly or partly satisfactory, but, in any case, should at the very least offer the clinical supervisor a 'springboard' for her own thoughts. The expert players in this game will only offer their contribution once the supervisee has finished speaking. Past champions have learnt to say nothing more than 'that sounds fairly logical to me, why don't you look it up in a book for next time, and see if you had it right all along'.

The more advanced – and professionally secure – player will, of course, make her own visit to the library and be able to offer a more informed opinion at the next meeting. One positive outcome of playing this game at the advanced level, is that no one actually loses. Information is usually gained by at least one or both pari-ties; the supervisor does not lose face and the supervisee is left feeling that he is in the hands of a concerned professional. The game can be completely avoided however, should the supervisor wish it, by careful use of the phrase 'I'm sorry, but I do not have any idea at all about that issue, would you like to look it up, and we can talk about it in depth, next time.'

Supervisor Game 3: 'Poor Me': This is a particularly useful game for the extra-busy and/or disorganised supervisor. It can be played whenever either party feels that the supervisor has failed to meet her agreed responsibilities. This can include being late in attending a clinical supervision session, or having to cancel the session at short notice. It can also be played whenever the supervisor is distracted during the clinical supervision, or appears to have something other than the supervisee's material on her mind. This game can be of most use to the supervisor when the supervisee wishes to challenge her for breaching their supervisory contract.

The main purpose of this game is to allow the supervisee to feel some sympathy for his supervisor which in itself, may prevent him from expressing disappointment, frustration or even anger to the supervisor due to her inadequate attention to his supervisory needs. Expert players can manage to not only arouse the supervisee's sympathy, but also feel fully ashamed of themselves for even daring to raise the issue, at one and the same time. The object of the game is for the clinical supervisor to attempt to rebuff any complaint – or even the merest suggestion that the clinical supervisee is unhappy – with a phrase that suggests that were she not so busy/important/as senior/popular or in demand, etc., then the supervisor would have lots of time to attend to the needs of her supervisee.

The supervisor can lose the game in one of two main ways:

1   The supervisor apologises for her failure to meet her supervisory obligations and does whatever she can to ensure that these are met in future.
2   The supervisee retorts with a polite comment to the effect that he appreciates that his supervisor is an extremely busy/important/senior/popular and/or in-demand person. He also appreciates, however, that she has an obligation in regard to offering him clinical supervision, and he would be grateful if she could do what she can to see that it is met, without delay or disruption.

8

Moving On – Groupwork and Endings in Clinical Supervision

Key issues in this chapter

- The advantages and disadvantages of group supervision
- Facilitated group supervision
- Peer group supervision
- The sixth stage of a supervisee's development
- Ending clinical supervision

Practising clinical supervision in groups

I will begin this brief overview of clinical supervision in groups by discussing some of the more important considerations for supervisors. I will then outline some forms of group supervision likely to be of most interest to nurses and conclude with a summary of the main advantages of conducting clinical supervision in groups – together with some common problems.

What is a clinical supervision group?

I use the term *supervision group* to describe a gathering of at least three people (one supervisor and two supervisees – or three supervisees alone, in the case of peer supervision) and up to a maximum of five people. I have yet to find a 'foolproof' method of determining the 'best' maximum number for a clinical supervision group but there are important factors to be considered when deciding on the size of the group, and these include:

THE EXPERIENCE AND SKILLS OF THE GROUP SUPERVISOR

Managing a group of supervisees will always be more difficult and require more skill on the part of the supervisor than she will need when working with an individual supervisee. Not only will the supervisor need to retain more information in her head, at any one time, she will also need to demonstrate greater skills of time management and group co-ordination, to ensure that each member is given a regular and, roughly, equal opportunity to participate. She will need to develop skills of encouragement to ensure that the more reticent members are not allowed to 'fade into the background', and skills of people-management to ensure that the more obstreperous members are not allowed free reign to dominate the proceedings.

THE TIME AVAILABLE

Time is an important factor when considering clinical supervision in a group. It will invariably be in short supply, both in terms of how much time the nursing organisation can allow for the process, and how much the participants themselves will be able to spare in order to attend. The group supervisor will need to ensure that each supervisee receives a regular and adequate amount of time to present his material and balance this concern against the inevitably limited time available to the group. It is not uncommon for supervision groups to be held for one and a half hours duration. If the supervisor wished to allow half an hour for each supervisee to present at each session, then she would need to limit the group size to three, and pro-rata, according to the desired presentation time and the time available for the group.

THE CAPACITY OF THE GROUP MEMBERS TO ATTEND REGULARLY

The supervisor who plans to run a large group, in the hope that it will prove more cost-effective and time-effective than a smaller one, could find herself regretting it, if not all of the members are able to attend all of the planned sessions. The bigger the group, the more chance there will be of absences from the sessions. An important factor in the survival of a clinical supervision group will be the capacity of its members to 'gel' together. Consistency of members' attendance, especially in the early life of the group, will often be crucial to its survival.

THE AVAILABILITY AND SIZE OF ROOMS

The room size is also important to consider because the whole group should be able to sit together in comfort, with a reasonable amount of space between the chairs. I prefer to lay out the seating for group supervision in a circular, or horse-shoe arrangement, which in itself demands a larger room than would be needed if the participants were to sit around a table. This latter arrangement should be avoided at all costs, in my view, even if the lack of a suitably large room means restricting the group to a small number or abandoning the idea altogether.

For these reasons alone, I recommend that the number of clinical supervisees in any one group should not exceed five. I also suggest that until a supervisor is considerably experienced in this work that she considers facilitating groups of no more than three supervisees together at any one time.

Two forms of supervision in groups

There are two basic forms of clinical group supervision that I wish to discuss here:

- Facilitated group supervision
- Peer group supervision

FACILITATED GROUP SUPERVISION

I use the term *facilitated group supervision* to refer to any clinical supervision session conducted by an approved clinical nurse supervisor for more than two supervisees together at any one time. The actual process of facilitated group supervision can take a number of different forms and which one takes precedence will often depend upon the clinical training of the supervisor and the supervisory requirements and therapeutic orientation of the supervisees. Carroll (1996) suggests that two main forms of facilitated group supervision are when:

1   A supervisor, designated as leader of the group, works with individuals within a group setting.
2   There is a designated leader but the group process within supervision is used as a learning focus.

I feel strongly that, except with the possible exception of those nurses specialising in certain forms of counselling and psychotherapy, there is no obvious place for the *exclusive* use of group dynamics in the clinical supervision of nurses. Used carefully and skilfully, however, such a focus can offer the potential for new learning, particularly with more experienced supervisees.

My own tendency is to incorporate a range of opportunities for supervisory learning into a repertoire of interventions that the group supervisor can use as and when she considers them to be appropriate and in keeping with the group's position and needs. Hawkins and Shohet (1989) feel that the group supervisor should ensure that any dynamics present between the supervisees (perhaps strongly positive or negative feelings or blatant criticism from one supervisee, or a section of the group, to another section or individual) are not left unacknowledged. They believe that an awareness of the group dynamics is an essential part of the learning process for supervisees, and that it is the group supervisor's task to bring them into awareness so that they can be attended to and learnt from, without allowing them to become the main focus of the group.

When the group supervisor is intending to work directly *with* the individual supervisees, rather than *through* the group itself, as she might when focusing on the group dynamics, there is no reason for her to feel restricted to conducting what amounts to nothing more than individual supervision with other people 'eavesdropping'.

PEER GROUP SUPERVISION

Gomersall (1997) has defined the *peer group* as:

> a group of people of similar status who are engaged in a similar line of work or in a co-operative project, who set aside regular committed time to examine the nature of the task and its effective accomplishment, and also examine those strengths and vulnerabilities – both as a group and as individuals – which may assist or inhibit the performance of the task. (Gomersall, 1997: 108)

Gomersall feels that the main advantage of the peer supervision group '. . . is in the enhancing of the efficiency of the work'. I believe that this aim should not be considered as an exclusive claim of the peer supervision group, but rather one that should be high on the list of priorities of all forms of group supervision and, indeed, clinical supervision generally in whatever form.

Enhanced efficiency in the nursing work will not, in itself, be an automatic by-product of peer group supervision. On the contrary, peer supervision groups that are not developed with considerable foresight and planning and that are not carefully managed and maintained throughout their existence will, at best, leave the participants feeling no more enhanced in skills and knowledge than they were at the outset and, at worst, leave them feeling professionally insecure, discouraged and reluctant to participate in future group activities.

Gomersall suggests that enhanced efficiency in the work, through peer group supervision, is, in fact, dependent upon a number of key factors which I have adapted to the purpose of nursing:

- The nurse's level of skill and knowledge.
- The nurse's level of morale related to his work.
- The nurse's sense of identity within his employing organisation.
- The quality of the nurse's working relationships with his peers.
- The quality of the nurse's working relationships with those senior to him in the professional hierarchy.
- The quality of the nurse's working relationships with those junior to him in the professional hierarchy.

The peer supervision group would appear, then, to have a dual-purpose of:

- Offering opportunities for the safe and positive sharing of ideas, skills, techniques and nursing knowledge.
- Offering opportunities for recognition of the relationship between the nurse's positive feelings of 'belonging' to, and of being 'valued' by, the nursing organisation and his capacity and enthusiasm to increase his skills and knowledge.

Peer supervision groups work best when they observe strict guidelines in terms of their purpose and function. Peer supervision group members should concern themselves with the *narrower perspectives* in no less a way than they would do for individual clinical supervision and I would advise the formulation of, and adherence to, a set of contractual guidelines at the outset. In addition to achieving a consensus on the duration and frequency of the group, the members should be very clear about what is its purpose and what is not. Peer supervision groups tend to work least well, and can often fail, if they are considered to have been imposed by senior management (Weiner and Caldwell, 1984) and/or if members attempt to use them for personal therapy (Kanas, 1986).

Advantages and disadvantages of clinical supervision in groups

Group supervision can appear to be a very attractive option for nurses when viewed from both the 'extented' and 'restricted' viewpoints, as described in Chapter 3. Although group supervision does have a part to play in addressing the problems faced by nursing organisations who are seeking to provide clinical supervision for large numbers of supervisees, it would be misleading to suggest that group supervision should always be seen as the primary method of choice. I see group and individual (one-to-one) supervision as different modes, both with their own unique qualities and potential drawbacks. It is important to suggest too, that group supervision should, ideally, be the choice of the supervisee rather than his only option. Unfortunately, because of its cost-effective nature and the relative scarcity of skilled supervisors, group supervision has a tendency to become the 'Hobson's Choice' of methods in some nursing organisations.

On learning from the supervisee

My own experience as both a clinical supervisor and supervisee includes many hours spent working in groups, large and small, both facilitated and 'peer'. In writing this section I have drawn not only from that experience but also from the experiences of five 'nurse-fellows' working in higher education, for whom I acted as group supervisor. Some of those nurses were given their first 'taste' of clinical supervision in that group, and others had been supervised elsewhere, both individually and in groups. They were kind enough to offer me their thoughts on the process and value of clinical supervision in a group, and I am pleased to be able to present their insightful comments, as an adjunct to my own views.

Some advantages of clinical supervision groups
INCREASED COST-EFFECTIVENESS
All clinical supervision groups will allow for the supervision of at least 100 per cent (and often 200 or 300 per cent) more nurses by the same supervisor, but with only around a 50 or 60 per cent increase in the time required to do so.

INCREASED POTENTIAL FOR THE GENERATION OF NEW AND ORIGINAL
IDEAS

Three heads can sometimes be better than two and so on.

> I supervise a group of nursing home practitioners and they've all
> got similar patients and similar issues, and they all have experience
> around working in a particular organisation. The supervisees often
> bring individual issues to that group and members will use their wider
> experience to add something to the overall supervision process. (Nurse-
> fellow)

INCREASED OPPORTUNITIES TO EXPLORE SUPERVISION TECHNIQUES

These can include role-play, psychodrama and other 'experiential'
exercises that would be impracticable in individual supervision.

INCREASED POTENTIAL FOR LEARNING FROM THE WORK AND
EXPERIENCES OF OTHERS

> Even when you've got a supervision group consisting of nurses working
> with the same patient group, the supervisees will have different views
> on how to work with those patients and that can be very valuable.
> (Nurse-fellow)

AN INCREASED SENSE OF 'COLLEGIALITY'

This may come from taking opportunities to be of assistance to
fellow nurse supervisees by using one's own nursing experiences
and knowledge for the benefit of others.

AN INCREASED SENSE OF SUPPORT

Learning to share difficulties and failures with others can offer the
supervisee important opportunities to take risks, test confidenti-
alities and develop trust.

> Sometimes, when someone brings an issue to the group it may be
> different from another person's issue but many of the people in the
> group will be able to relate it to their own work and experiences.
> (Nurse-fellow)

GAINING A SENSE OF 'TOGETHERNESS'

This can result from the supervisees' experience of sharing
anxieties, and aspirations with nurses at a similar stage of experience and knowledge or those working with a similar patient group.

> We all knew that there were common issues when we decided to have
> supervision and that's why we set the group up. We were all talking

about issues that were common to ourselves and said: 'Wouldn't it be good if we could do this in a more structured way.' (Nurse-fellow)

GAINING A SENSE OF INDEPENDENCE FROM THE SUPERVISOR

Group supervisees can learn to rely more on other group members (peers) and themselves for solutions to problems, rather than the supervisor. In this way, they become less dependent upon one particular person and develop an understanding that supervisors are not 'special' or 'infallible'.

Some disadvantages of clinical supervision groups

With any method, there is always some potential for negative consequences to arise through its use. Group supervision is no exception and I have included a few potential difficulties that can arise in group supervision, in order that both supervisors and supervisees can be forewarned – and thus forearmed.

DISAGREEMENTS ABOUT THE ALLOCATION OF TIME FOR SUPERVISORY ATTENTION

If group members do not feel that they are receiving an equal amount of time to present material and receive feedback, it can result in members becoming disheartened and eventually leaving the group.

SCAPEGOATING

This can occur when 'weaker' members of the group are allowed to accept negative and hostile feelings, such as anger, blame, anxiety and disappointment which belong to others in the group or the group as a whole. This can frequently result in the loss of capable members and disruption of the group.

LESS OPPORTUNITY TO PRESENT MATERIAL

Nurses with a larger than average caseload (or patient group) may have less opportunity to present all of their clinical material than those nurses in the group with a smaller caseload.

BREACHES OF CONFIDENTIALITY

As the group numbers increase, the possibility of confidential information being 'leaked' may also increase.

FORMATION OF 'SUB-GROUPS' AND 'RIVAL CAMPS'
This is more likely to occur only in the larger supervision groups. It can lead to information being shared outside the group and the consequential difficulty of certain information being known only to a select few.

DISRUPTIONS CAUSED BY THE LATENESS AND/OR ABSENTEEISM OF MEMBERS
The larger the group is, the more potential there will be for lateness and absenteeism. If this occurs early in the life of the group, it may never have the opportunity to 'form' properly. Regular attenders may also become disheartened by persistent latecomers or absentees and find it difficult to feel comfortable and 'safe' about presenting.

Parting in such sweet sorrow – the end phase of clinical supervision

Although clinical supervision can be a process that occurs throughout the nurse's entire professional life, the possibility that a particular supervisory relationship will end, at some point, must be seriously considered and preferably well in advance of the event. In addition, it is always prudent for supervisors to think about procedures that may assist the closure process and ensure that it occurs as positively as possible, ideally, from before any supervisory relationship even begins.

Below, I offer three main reasons why a clinical supervision relationship may need to be brought to a close:

1 Reasons unconnected with the nature of the supervisory relationship. These allow future time in which to plan a suitable ending, and include:
   (a) The supervisor leaving her current post and the nursing organisation itself.
   (b) The supervisor changing roles within the organisation, affecting her capacity to offer supervision to this (and possibly any other) supervisee.
   (c) The supervisor choosing to discontinue her role for other professional and/or personal reasons.
   (d) The supervisee leaving his current post and the nursing organisation.

    (e) The supervisee changing roles within the organisation, affecting his capacity to receive clinical supervision from his current supervisor.

2   Reasons connected to a breakdown in the supervisory relationship. These may or may not allow future time in which to plan a suitable ending, and include:

    (a) A 'personality clash' between supervisor and supervisee.

    (b) The supervisor's method, style and/or model of supervision being unacceptable to the supervisee or incompatible with his current needs.

    (c) The supervisor becoming concerned that the supervisee is practising 'unsafely', unethically or, in some other way, improperly and choosing to discontinue his supervision.

3   Reasons for the sudden termination of the supervisory relationship. These will mean the termination of the supervision without the opportunity to plan a suitable ending, and include:

    (a) The sudden death of the supervisor or her supervisee.

    (b) The suspension or dismissal from duty of the supervisor or her supervisee.

Procedures for discontinuing clinical supervision

When the supervisor and supervisee both agree that the supervision sessions should be terminated, it is important that this is done by agreement, and by following a pre-agreed system. It is always important to follow such procedures and essential to do so when the reasons for termination may be considered in any way acrimonious, debatable or enforced.

What form termination procedures should take, largely depends on what is agreed as right and proper by both the clinical supervisor and her supervisee. However it will usually be important to identify exactly what should be done with regard to certain specific factors of the supervision process including:

- The amount of notice (usually stated as a number of weeks or sessions) to be given by either party should they intend to cease from providing or receiving clinical supervision.
- The reason for the decision.
- The names of any additional person to be notified of the cancellation of the supervisory arrangement.
- The circumstances under which the person above will be notified of the reasons for cancellation of the supervisory arrangement.

Think about . . . two ways to terminate clinical supervision

Read the two short scenarios below and consider what the consequences of each might be. Consider especially:

a) What the relationship between supervisor and supervisee might be like now and how it may be affected in the long-term.

b) What the effect might be on the supervisor's professional reputation.

SCENARIO 1

Supervisor: I am concerned about the way things have been going lately.

Supervisee: Are you? I think things are going OK but I'm sure that you know best.

Supervisor: I probably do, at least about this, and I think perhaps it would be best if we stopped the supervision sessions.

Supervisee: Why do you want to do that? I'm just getting into it!

Supervisor: You tend to use the time more for personal therapy than a clinical supervision. It's a misuse of the time and of skills and experience. I think you are behaving most unprofessionally by asking me to work in that way.

Supervisee: I totally disagree, there's nothing wrong with bringing my personal experiences into supervision. Any half-decent supervisor would not expect me to keep my personal and professional life totally separate. I expected someone like you to say that. You're so rigid in your thinking that I'm surprised you don't issue a script when I arrive each time.

Supervisor: We have obviously reached a point in our working relationship that will be difficult for us to recover from. I suggest that we stop the supervision immediately and that you look for a new supervisor.

Supervisee: Fine. But don't expect me not to complain about this! [*The supervisee exits hurriedly while the supervisor considers herself lucky to not be abused further by such an uncouth individual!*]

SCENARIO 2

Supervisor: I wondered if we could not get into the specific issues of your supervision straight away today, but talk instead, about the sessions themselves for a bit?

Supervisee: OK, but why would you want to do that?

Supervisor: Thanks. Well, I am concerned about the way the sessions have been going lately . . .

Supervisee: What are you concerned about, in particular?

Supervisor: There have been several times, recently, when you have preferred to talk more about your home-life than your work – do you think that's a fair assessment?

Supervisee: It's not always the case, but I can see that I have perhaps not kept the issues completely separate, it's not always that easy to do, as you must know.

Supervisor: I think there will inevitably be some overlapping of the two strands of your life in some of things we will discuss. What I have been most concerned about, is that you seem to talk less about the situations at work directly and much more about how work is affecting you at home and in your personal relationships.

Supervisee: I enjoy talking about my personal problems to you, I've never been able to open up to anyone else like this before!

Supervisor: Well, I find that flattering but my task is to help you with work-related issues and that's not happening as much as I hoped it would. If I am to do the best thing by you I can't let the sessions continue along these lines. My problem is that I'm not really convinced that it will be easy for us to revert to purely work-based sessions, in the future.

Supervisee: I take your point. Perhaps it's best if we stopped then? I've benefited over the past few weeks but perhaps I should find a supervisor that I don't want to use as a therapist.

Supervisor: We agreed when we made our supervision contract that we would have one more session after deciding to stop the supervision. It will give us time to say goodbye properly and hopefully for us to look for an alternative supervisor for you. Shall we meet as usual next time then?

Supervisee: Yes, I'll see you in four weeks, for our final session. [*The supervisor opens the door for the supervisee, who then wishes her well before leaving, quietly.*]

Issues and concerns about ending clinical supervision

I once had a colleague who, when meeting a new group of students, would endeavour to 'tune into' their anxieties around embarking on their new adventure with the phrase 'beginnings can be difficult'. As valid a maxim as that might be for understanding some of the difficulties with relationships, I am yet to be convinced that endings are not even harder. To stop doing something that we are familiar and comfortable with, no matter how stressful it may have been at times, can be very traumatic and unsettling. Even when moving on seems like the best option, we may not be sure of what might be around the corner and might find ourselves wondering if staying put – wearing the same old comfortable sweater rather than trying on the new suit – might not be the wisest, and safest course of action. But, sometimes, the safest way is not best way. Also, even when we choose not to change our situation, a change may well be forced upon us. No matter how it hard it becomes, we then have to try to deal with it in a way that leaves us feeling good about moving forward and not looking back – no matter how tempting that may seem.

Carroll (1996: 112) has detailed a range of issues that can be generated for the supervisee (and perhaps for the supervisor, as well) when a clinical supervision arrangement comes to an end. All of these issues are ones that might arise for an individual confronted with the 'ending' of a significant aspect of his life outside clinical supervision. I have adapted Carroll's original list slightly, and used the prefix 'a sense of . . . ', to indicate that although these feelings may be around for many of us when something stops or changes or ends; whether it will be a reality for us depends, often, on our personal development, practical situation, what are our immediate plans, what is our current level of social support and why the ending occurred at all.

WHAT WE MAY EXPERIENCE WHEN A RELATIONSHIP ENDS
- A sense of . . . having to 'grow up'.
- A sense of . . . being separated.
- A sense of . . . being abandoned.
- A sense of . . . being alone.
- A sense of . . . needing someone else in our lives.
- A sense of . . . not being good enough.
- A sense of . . . being let down.
- A sense of . . . finding it hard to trust others.
- A sense of . . . having to make other choices.
- A sense of . . . loss.

There are also factors that may have a bearing on how the supervisee is affected by the ending of the clinical supervision process. Two important ones raised by Stoltenberg and Delworth (1987) are:

The gender of the supervisee can be important in determining those that will find it easier to end a relationship, than to begin it, according to Stoltenberg and Delworth. They draw on the work of Gilligan (1982) who suggests that women find it more difficult to end a relationship and men find it more difficult to begin one. Stoltenberg and Delworth use this work to suggest that female supervisees may be more reluctant to end a period of supervision and male supervisees may not take the ending 'seriously' – or 'finally' – enough and look for another way to have an on-going relationship with the supervisor.

My own view is that there is unlikely to be any benefit to the supervisor from assuming that both of the above factors should be used as anything other than very simple guidelines to the possible

responses of their supervisees on termination of the clinical supervision. Different supervisees are likely to act in different ways,
depending upon the circumstances, their experiences and current
professional situation. The astute supervisor will get to know her
supervisee well and use that understanding as a guide to how he
may respond to the ending of the professional relationship.

The stage of professional development that the supervisee is at when
the supervision ends is important because it may affect the way in
which the supervisee responds to the ending itself. Supervisees
still in the 'beginning phase' of clinical supervision when it is
terminated may lose trust in their supervisor, but often find it
easier to bond with a new supervisor than a supervisee who is in
the 'middle phase' of his clinical supervision. This supervisee is
also likely to have a sense of mistrust associated not only to his
current supervisor but also with others offering to supervise him
in the future. In this respect, he is likely to be more cynical than
the beginner.

DEVELOPMENT STAGE 6 – CALM AND COLLEGIALITY
Clinical supervision terminated when the supervisee is at the final
stage of his professional development is likely to be the least
traumatic of all. Very experienced supervisees, according to
Stoltenberg and Delworth (1987), may find it possible to see the
ending as a parting of friends, with no 'unfinished business' or
'bad feelings'.

When he reaches this, final, stage of professional development,
the supervisee will be demonstrating a strong professional identity
of his own. He will know what sort of nurse he is, what particular
forms of nursing care he enjoys and excels at, and which ones he is
less expert in or enjoys least. The supervisor may find herself
listening to the supervisee's plans for the future and his views on
the developments of nursing in a wider context, perhaps as he
reviews the effects of organisational and political decisions effecting nursing care both locally and nationally. Something that the
supervisor will notice, perhaps above all, is that her supervisee will
have become much more of a 'settled', calmer and less potentially
disruptive individual than the one he was during the fifth stage of
his development. He will, in fact, be regularly displaying a great
deal of respect for his colleagues, including his supervisor, and if
he disagrees with the views of others, he will be able to say so in a
reasoned and informed way that is markedly different from the

argumentative and disagreeable style he might have employed during the earlier stages of his development. The supervisee may also be expressing a desire to be involved in the clinical supervision of other nurses, either as a 'peer' or facilitator in his own right. Typical characteristics of the supervisee at this stage (as outlined by Stolenberg and Delworth, 1987) can include:

- Personal autonomy
- Insightful awareness
- Personal security
- Stable motivation
- Awareness of professional strengths and weaknesses

Many experienced supervisors will consider themselves fortunate, indeed, to be able to see the end of a period of clinical supervision for a supervisee who has reached the sixth stage of his professional development. Although this may not happen frequently, when it does it can be as if she is saying goodbye to a mature and experienced colleague of similar professional standing. The sense of personal autonomy, insightful awareness and personal security that her supervisee should be exuding when he reaches this stage of development, will help both to feel that the ending is apt and 'safe'.

Using the ending of supervision to the benefit of the supervisee

Carroll (1996) suggests a process of termination in clinical supervision that offers a pragmatic and positive three-stage approach to ending supervision in a way that can be regarded as constructive and forward-looking by the supervisee. I have outlined my adaptation of the process below, together with thoughts on how nursing supervisees may best use it.

SUMMARISING PROGRESS

The supervisor can encourage her supervisee to consolidate the learning that has taken place within their relationship and the psychological 'distance' that they have travelled together, as a way of allowing the supervisee to regard the time spent as constructive and not 'wasted'. This can involve:

- Reviewing what has happened over the course of the supervision period.

- Evaluating the strengths and weaknesses of the supervision arrangement.
- Discussing what particular interventions of the supervisor worked best for her supervisee.
- Evaluating the progress of the supervisee in his nursing care of the patients presented and how this may have developed.

DISCUSSING HOW CHANGES WILL BE MAINTAINED
There is a golden opportunity, here, for the supervisee to look forward to the next stage in his nursing career and/or development. By focusing on the future, the relationship coming to an end can be seen as an important stepping-stone towards the supervisee's ultimate destination in his nursing career.

ACHIEVING A SENSE OF CLOSURE
For me, 'closure' is about ensuring that the relationship is clearly seen, by both parties, as completely over. If a relationship – whether personal or professional – is closed properly there should be few concerns over 'unfinished business' and a consequential need for one or both participants to attempt to reinstate it at some later date, or to never fully 'let go' and remain in contact in some subtle way thereafter. This might mean the supervisor talking with the supervisee about what the ending means to both of them, and even expressing a sense of loss – even of missing the other person – if this is honest and appropriate. To ensure that the clinical supervision relationship closes properly, the supervisor and supervisee might wish to:

- Spend some time at the last meeting 'rounding off' the work previously discussed and clarifying how the supervision of any on-going work of the supervisee will be provided.
- Spend some time at the last meeting recounting what the other person has meant to them (as a supervisor or supervisee) and by stating what each has gained, professionally, from knowing the other person.
- Say 'goodbye' and 'thank you' both literally, and in the form of a hand-shake.

When a supervision that has lasted for a reasonable length of time, during which learning and professional development has occurred and in which the supervisor and her supervisee have grown to respect each other as professionals is over, either or both of the participants could be forgiven for thinking that they have left behind them something that will be irreplaceable. They will, no doubt, have experienced something that is very special and probably unique. An experience that is different from any personal relationship or nursing relationship that they might ever have. They should both treasure it and be aware of its value. But they should not assume that it is irreplaceable. Like most important experiences in life, supervision can be found in different places and with different people and the experience can be no less valuable or special or unique, than the ones that were closed along the supervisee's way. What it will almost certainly be, though, is different. And the 'difference' in supervision, just as in life, is often the very thing that can make it all worthwhile.

References

Argyle, M. (1992) *The Social Psychology of Everyday Life*. London: Routledge.

August, O. (1997) 'Marathon across Sahara lures the English patient', *The Times*, 29 March, p. 13.

Bent, A. (1992) 'The statutory basis to the role of the supervisor', in English National Board, *Preparation of Supervisors of Midwives*. London: English National Board.

Berne, E. (1964) *Games People Play*. London: Grove Press.

Bion, W. (ed.) (1980) *Bion in New York and São Paulo*. Perthshire: Clunie Press.

Bion, W. (1974) 'Brazilian Lectures 1', in P. Casement (1985) *On Learning from the Patient*. London: Tavistock Publications.

Bond, M. and Holland, S. (1998) *Skills of Clinical Supervision for Nurses*. Buckingham: Open University Press.

Boseley, S. (1997) 'Nurses claim victory over local pay', *The Guardian*, 7 February, p. 7.

Boyd, J. (1978) *Counselor Supervision*. Indiana: Accelerated Development Inc.

Bromberg, P.M. (1982) 'The supervision process and parallel process in psychoanalysis', *Contemporary Psychoanalysis*, 18 (1), 93–111.

Buber, M. (1958) *I and Thou*, Tr. R.G. Smith. Edinburgh: T.T Clarke.

Burns, M.E. (1958) 'The historical development of the process of casework supervision as seen in the professional literature of social work'. PhD Dissertation, University of Chicago.

Butterworth, T., Carson, J., White, E., Jeacock, J., Clements, A. and Bishop, V. (1997) *It Is Good To Talk: An Evaluation of Clinical Supervision and Mentorship in England and Scotland*. Manchester: University of Manchester.

Carroll, M. (1996) *Counselling Supervision: Theory, Skills and Practice*. London: Cassell.

Community Psychiatric Nurses' Association (1989) *Clinical Practice Issues for CPNs*. London: CPNA Publications.

Daloz, L.A. (1986) *Effective Teaching and Mentoring: Realising the Transformational Power of Adult Learning Experiences*. San Francisco: Jossey-Bass.

Department of Health (1993) *A Vision for the Future*. London: National Health Service Management Executive.

Dimond, B. (1998) 'Legal aspects of clinical supervision 2: professional accountability', *British Journal of Nursing*, 7 (8): 487–9.

Doehrman, M.J. (1976) 'Parallel processes in supervision and psychotherapy', *Bulletin of the Menninger Clinic*, 40: 9–104.

East, P. (1995) 'The mentoring relationship', in R.B. Ellis, R.J. Gates and N. Kenworthy (eds), *Interpersonal Communication in Nursing: Theory and Practice*. Edinburgh: Churchill Livingstone.

Ellis, R.B. (1995) 'Defining communication', in R.B. Ellis, R.J. Gates and N. Kenworthy (eds), *Interpersonal Communication in Nursing: Theory and Practice*. Edinburgh: Churchill Livingstone.

Evans, D. (1997) 'Supervision today: the psychoanalytic legacy', in G. Shipton (ed.), *Supervision of Psychotherapy and Counselling: Making a Place to Think*. Buckingham: Open University Press.

Farrington, A. (1996) 'Clinical supervision: UKCC must be more proactive', *British Journal of Nursing*, 5 (12): 716.

Faugier, J. (1992) 'The supervisory relationship', in C.A. Butterworth and J. Faugier (eds), *Clinical Supervision and Mentorship in Nursing*. London: Chapman & Hall.

Faugier, J. (1996) 'Clinical supervision and mental health nursing', in T. Sandford and K. Gournay (eds), *Perspectives in Mental Health Nursing*. London: Baillière Tindall.

Freud, S. (1910) 'The future prospects of psychoanalytic therapy', *Standard Edition*, Vol. 11. London: Hogarth Press and the Institute of Psychoanalysis.

Freud, S. (1912) 'A note on the unconscious in psychoanalysis', *Standard Edition*, Vol. 12. London: Hogarth Press and the Institute of Psychoanalysis.

Freud, S. (1914) 'Remembering, repeating, working through', *Standard Edition*, Vol. 12. London: Hogarth Press and the Institute of Psychoanalysis.

Freud, S. (1915) 'Observations on transference love', *Standard Edition*, Vol. 12. London: Hogarth Press and the Institute of Psychoanalysis.

Freud, S. (1915) 'The unconscious', *Standard Edition*, Vol. 14. London: Hogarth Press and the Institute of Psychoanalysis.

Freud, S. (1927) 'The future of an illusion', *Standard Edition*, Vol. 22. London: Hogarth Press and the Institute of Psychoanalysis.

Friedman, D. and Kaslow, N.J. (1986) 'The development of professional identity in psychotherapists: six stages in the supervision process', in F.W. Kaslow (ed.), *Supervision and Training Models, Dilemmas and Challenges*. New York: Haworth Press.

Gilligan, C. (1982) *In a Different Voice: Psychological Theory and Women's Development*. Harvard: Harvard University Press.

Gomersall, J. (1997) 'Peer group supervision', in G. Shipton (ed.), *Supervision of Psychotherapy and Counselling: Making a Place to Think*. Buckingham: Open University Press.

Guardian, The (1996) 'Nurse interfered with life support', 4th October, p. 10.

Hawkins, P. (1985) 'Humanistic psychotherapy supervision: a conceptual framework', *Self and Society: European Journal of Humanistic Psychology*, 13 (2): 69–77.

Hawkins, P. and Shohet, R. (1989) *Supervision in the Helping Professions*. Buckingham: Open University Press.

Heron, J. (1975) *Six Category Intervention Analysis*. Guildford: University of Surrey.

Hobson, R.F. (1985) *Forms of Feeling: The Heart of Psychotherapy*. London: Tavistock Publications.

Hora, T. (1957) 'Contribution to the phenomenology of the supervisory process', *American Journal of Psychotherapy*, 11: 769–73.

Ivey, A.E. (1971) *Microcounselling: Innovation in Interview Training*. Illinois: Charles C. Thomas.

Ivey, A.E. and Simek-Downing, L. (1980) *Counselling and Psychotherapy Skills, Theories and Practice*. New Jersey: Prentice-Hall.

Kadushin, A. (1968) 'Games people play in supervision', *Social Work*, July.

Kadushin, A. (1992) *Supervision in Social Work*, 3rd edition. New York: Columbia University Press.

Kanas, N. (1986) 'Support groups for mental health staff and trainees', *International Journal of Group Psychotherapy*, 36: 279–96.

Keats, J. (1817) 'Letter to George and Thomas Keats', 21 December, in P. Casement (1985) *On Learning from the Patient*. London: Tavistock Publications.

Klauber, J. (1980) 'Formulating interpretations in clinical psychoanalysis', *International Journal of Psychoanalysis*, 61: 195–201.

Kohner, N. (1994) *Clinical Supervision in Practice*. London: Kings Fund Centre.

Leddick, G.R. and Bernard, J.M. (1980) 'The history of supervision: a critical review', *Counsellor Education and Supervision*, March, pp. 186–96.

Levinson, D. (1978) 'The seasons of a man's life', in P. East (1995) 'The mentoring relationship', in R.B. Ellis, R.J. Gates and N. Kenworthy (eds), *Interpersonal Communication in Nursing: Theory and Practice*. Edinburgh: Churchill Livingstone.

Lieberman, S. and Cobb, J.P. (1987a) 'The grammar of psychotherapy: a descriptive account', *British Journal of Psychiatry*, 151: 589–93.

Lieberman, S. and Cobb, J.P. (1987b) 'The grammar of psychotherapy: interactograms: three self monitoring instruments for audio tape feedback', *British Journal of Psychiatry*, 151: 594–601.

Loganbill, C., Hardy, E. and Delworth, U. (1982) 'Supervision, a conceptual model', *The Counselling Psychologist*, 10 (1): 3–42.

McFarlane, J. (1982) 'A charter for caring', *Journal of Advanced Nursing*, 1: 187–96.

McLeod, W.T. (ed.) (1987) *Collins Universal Dictionary of the English Language*. London: William Collins.

McNeill, B.W. and Worthen, V. (1989) 'The parallel process in psychotherapy supervision', *Professional Psychology: Research and Practice*, 20 (5): 329–33.

McQuail, D. (1984) *Communication*, 2nd edition. Harlow: Longman.

Maguire, P., Goldberg, D., Hyde, S., Jones, D., O'Dowd, T. and Roe, P. (1978) 'The value of feedback in teaching interviewing skills to medical', *Psychological Medicine*, 8: 695–704.

Meares, R. and Hobson, R.F. (1977) 'The persecutory therapist', *British Journal of Medical Psychology*, 50: 349–59.

Morrall, P. (1985) 'Social factors affecting communication', in R.B. Ellis, R.J. Gates and N. Kenworthy (eds), *Interpersonal Communication in Nursing: Theory and Practice*. Edinburgh: Churchill Livingstone.

Pesut, D.J. and Williams, C.A. (1990) 'The nature of clinical supervision in psychiatric nursing: a survey of clinical specialists', *Archives of Psychiatric Nursing*, 4 (3): 188–94.

Platt-Koch, J.M. (1986) 'Clinical supervision for psychiatric nurses', *Journal of Psychological Nursing*, 26 (1): 7–15.

Power, S. (1994a) 'A unique source of support and advice: the benefits of supervision in clinical practice', *Psychiatric Care*, 1 (3): 105–8.

Power, S. (1994b) 'Developing a constructive relationship: practical aspects of supervision', *Psychiatric Care*, 1 (4): 144–7.

Proctor, B. (1986) 'Supervision: a co-operative exercise in accountability', in M. Markham and M. Payne (eds), *Enabling and Ensuring*. Leicester: National Youth Bureau for Education in Youth and Community Work.

Reed, J. and Procter, S. (1993) *Nurse Education: A Reflective Approach*. Sevenoaks: Edward Arnold.

Rowntree, D. (1981) *A Dictionary of Education*. London: Harper & Row.

Schön, D.A. (1987) *Educating The Reflective Practitioner*. San Francisco: Jossey-Bass.

Searles, H. (1955) 'The informational value of the supervisor's emotional experiences', in *Collected Papers on Schizophrenia and Related Subjects*. London: Hogarth Press.

Shainberg, D. (1989) 'Teaching therapists to be with their clients', in P. Hawkins and R. Shohet (eds), *Supervision in the Helping Professions*. Buckingham: Open University Press.

Sloan, G. (1996) 'Clinical supervision: characteristics of a good supervisor', *Nursing Standard*, 12 (40): 42–6.

Stoltenberg, C.D. and Delworth, U. (1987) *Supervising Counsellors and Therapists*. San Francisco: Jossey Bass.

Swain, G. (1995) *Clinical Supervision: The Principles and Process*. London: Community Practitioners and Health Visitors Association.

UKCC (1996) *Position Statement on Clinical Supervision for Nursing and Health Visiting*. London: United Kingdom Central Council for Nursing, Midwifery and Health Visiting.

UKCC (1998) *Complaints About Professional Conduct*. London: United Kingdom Central Council for Nursing, Midwifery and Health Visiting.

Watzlawick, P., Beavin, J. and Jackson, D. (1967) *Pragmatics of Human Communication*. New York: Norton.

Weiner, M.F. and Caldwell, T. (1984) 'The process and impact of an ICU nurse support group', *International Journal of Psychiatry in Medicine*, 13: 47–55.

Wilkin, P. (1998a) *Clinical Supervision: The Rochdale Support and Development Model*. Rochdale: Rochdale Healthcare NHS Trust.

Wilkin, P. (1998b) 'Regeneration: a hermeneutic, phenomenological enquiry into the supportive experiences of community psychiatric nurses in clinical supervision'. Unpublished MA dissertation, Sheffield University.

Wilkin, P. (1999) 'Extract from a letter to a Pal', private correspondence with the author. Reproduced with written permission.

Williams, I.D.I. (1992) 'Supervision: a new word is desperately needed', *Counselling*, May.

Index